MAJOR CHRONIC DISEASES

This new series is designed to meet the growing demand for current, accessible information about the increasingly popular wellness approach to personal health. The result of a collaborative effort by a highly professional writing, editorial, and publishing team, the *Wellness* series consists of 16 volumes, each on a single topic. Each volume in this attractively produced series combines original material with carefully selected readings, relevant statistical data, and illustrations. The series objectives are to increase awareness of the value of a wellness approach to personal health and to help the reader become a more informed consumer of health-related information. Employing a critical thinking approach, each volume includes a variety of assessment tools, discusses basic concepts, suggests key questions, and provides the reader with a list of resources for further exploration.

James K. Jackson	Wellness: AIDS, STD, & Other Communicable Diseases
Richard G. Schlaadt	Wellness: Alcohol Use & Abuse
Richard G. Schlaadt	Wellness: Drugs, Society, & Behavior
Robert E. Kime	Wellness: Environment & Health
Gary Klug & Janice Lettunich	Wellness: Exercise & Physical Fitness
James D. Porterfield & Richard St. Pierre	Wellness: Healthful Aging
Robert E. Kime	Wellness: The Informed Health Consumer
Paula F. Ciesielski	Wellness: Major Chronic Diseases
Robert E. Kime	Wellness: Mental Health
Judith S. Hurley	Wellness: Nutrition & Health
Robert E. Kime	Wellness: Pregnancy, Childbirth, & Parenting
David C. Lawson	Wellness: Safety & Accident Prevention
Randall R. Cottrell	Wellness: Stress Management
Richard G. Schlaadt	Wellness: Tobacco & Health
Randall R. Cottrell	Wellness: Weight Control
Judith S. Hurley & Richard G. Schlaadt	Wellness: The Wellness Life-Style

MAJOR CHRONIC DISEASES

Paula F. Ciesielski

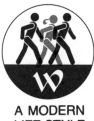

WELLNESS

A MODERN
LIFE-STYLE
LIBRARY

The Dushkin Publishing Group, Inc./Sluice Dock, Guilford, CT 06437

To my mother, Barbara Ford

Library of Congress Catalog Card Number: 91–072190
Manufactured in the United States of America
First Edition, First Printing
ISBN: 0–87967–873–9

Library of Congress Cataloging-in-Publication Data

Ciesielski, Paula F., Major Chronic Diseases (Wellness)
    1. Chronic diseases. I. Title. II. Series.
RA642.2   616   91–072190   ISBN 0–87967–873–9

Please see page 162 for credits.

The procedures and explanations given in this publication are based on research and consultation with medical and nursing authorities. To the best of our knowledge, these procedures and explanations reflect currently accepted medical practice; nevertheless, they cannot be considered absolute and universal recommendations. For individual application, treatment suggestions must be considered in light of the individual's health, subject to a doctor's specific recommendations. The authors and the publisher disclaim responsibility for any adverse effects resulting directly or indirectly from the suggested procedures, from any undetected errors, or from the reader's misunderstanding of the text.

PAULA F. CIESIELSKI

Dr. Paula F. Ciesielski is a staff physician at the University of Oregon Student Health Center. A native of Portland, Oregon, she received her B.S. in chemistry from the University of Puget Sound, Washington, and her M.D. from Oregon Health Sciences University. She practiced internal medicine and intensive care privately in conjunction with her father, who is also an M.D., before going on to the University of Oregon where she now actively pursues her interest in preventive medicine.

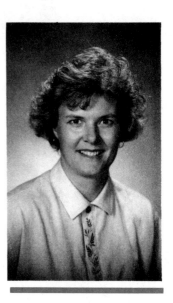

WELLNESS:
A Modern Life-Style Library

General Editors
Robert E. Kime, Ph.D.
Richard G. Schlaadt, Ed.D.

Authors
Paula F. Ciesielski, M.D.
Randall R. Cottrell, Ed.D.
Judith S. Hurley, M.S., R.D.
James K. Jackson, M.D.
Robert E. Kime, Ph.D.
Gary A. Klug, Ph.D.
David C. Lawson, Ph.D.
Janice Lettunich, M.S.
James D. Porterfield
Richard St. Pierre, Ph.D.
Richard G. Schlaadt, Ed.D.

Developmental Staff
Irving Rockwood, Program Manager
Paula Edelson, Series Editor
James D. Porterfield, Developmental Editor
Wendy Connal, Administrative Assistant
Jason J. Marchi, Editorial Assistant

Editing Staff
John S. L. Holland, Managing Editor
Elizabeth Jewell, Copy Editor
Diane Barker, Editorial Assistant
Mary L. Strieff, Art Editor
Robert Reynolds, Illustrator

Production and Design Staff
Brenda S. Filley, Production Manager
Whit Vye, Cover Design and Logo
Jeremiah B. Lighter, Text Design
Libra Ann Cusack, Typesetting Supervisor
Charles Vitelli, Designer
Meredith Scheld, Graphics Assistant
Steve Shumaker, Graphics Assistant
Lara M. Johnson, Graphics Assistant
Juliana Arbo, Typesetter
Richard Tietjen, Editorial Systems Analyst

A S A PHYSICIAN who specializes in the treatment of acute and chronic adult diseases, I see the consequences of life-style choices that lead to disease on a daily basis. This book is written in the hope that increased awareness of these choices will help the reader enhance his or her chance of leading a longer, healthier, life while avoiding the diseases discussed in the pages that follow.

These diseases, all of which are chronic, are different in many ways, but share several attributes. First, they are among the leading causes of death and disability throughout the industrialized world today. Second, they tend not to occur suddenly, as do many communicable diseases, but rather to develop slowly over a long period of time and then linger. For these reasons they have long been known as chronic diseases. Last, they are in many instances the product of life-style. For this reason, they are increasingly known as the "life-style diseases."

To be sure, such diseases are not solely the product of life-style. Genetics clearly plays a role in determining who succumbs, and even the healthiest life-style offers no guarantee against an inherited susceptibility to coronary heart disease or any of the other diseases discussed in this volume. But even among those who are genetically predisposed, changes in life-style can make a difference. And such changes, primarily in eating, smoking, and exercise habits, have been occurring. Most experts agree that such changes explain at least in part the steady reduction in mortality from heart disease and stroke that we have been observing since the 1960s. Now, more than ever, control over the factors that influence our health is in our own hands.

Like any effective health education program, the content of this book is designed to help you with three tasks that are central to any effective health education program. Factual descriptions of the various disorders provide the information needed to understand and identify the problem. Self-assessments and readings are provided to help with the task of assessing your own level of risk. Finally, there are a variety of practical suggestions to help you apply what you have learned. Much of this last type of material, including a plan for action, appears in the last chapter.

This is not a definitive work, but rather a place to begin. the central objective of this book is not to make you into an instant expert but to help you learn to *think critically* about the information on disease, health, and life-style with which all of us are bombarded almost daily. Only then will you be able to distinguish health fact from health myth, and only then will you be an informed health consumer.

I am grateful to James K. Jackson, Richard G. Schlaadt, and Robert E. Kime, all of the University of Oregon, for the opportunity to write this book. In addition, I would like to acknowledge the contribution of the two editors with whom I worked most closely, James D. Porterfield and Paula Edelson. Their expertise has made this book possible.

Beyond this, I am grateful to my parents, Peter S. and Barbara Ford, for being examples of loving human beings. My father is a remarkable physician, and it is to his credit that I chose his profession. My gratitude for my husband, Michael, goes beyond words. He was critic, encourager, computer expert, typist, and endless source of unconditional love. I would like to thank my children, Ann and Thomas, for their patience and love during the time this book was being written. I am also grateful to my extended family whose love and support is always with me and of which it is a privilege to be a part. Lastly, I would like to thank all the patients that have taught me about medicine and life over the years.

Paula F. Ciesielski
Eugene, OR

Contents

1

Coronary Heart Disease
Page 1

4

Diseases
of the Lung
Page 85

6

A Personal Plan of Action
Page 129

FIGURES

TABLES

Coronary Heart Disease

ADVANCES IN MEDICINE and public health over the last 100 years have had a significant impact on life expectancy and death rates in the United States. For example, in 1900 the average life expectancy for a white male was 48 years. [1] In 1990 life expectancy at birth for people born in the United States was 72 years for men, 79 years for women. [2]

Earlier in this century, many people died from diseases associated with infection and poor sanitation. Since 1900 the discovery and use of antibiotics and immunization serums, a significant reduction in infant and childhood death rates, and efforts to improve sanitation have all made substantial contributions to improving the health and life expectancy of most Americans. [3]

As a result, today over half of all deaths in the United States are caused by diseases of the heart and blood vessels. [4] Of all major chronic diseases, heart disease is the one most influenced by our life-style. It is ironic, then, that the leading fatal disease may be the disease most easily prevented by changes in our lifestyle.

Cardiovascular disease is the medical term for any disease of the heart (cardio) or blood vessels (vascular). The most common form of heart disease is **atherosclerosis**, a buildup of **cholesterol**, fat, and cellular debris within the lining of the victim's arteries. **Arteries** are the blood vessels that carry freshly oxygenated blood from the heart to the body's tissues. The buildup of deposits in the arteries, like rust in a pipe, narrows and, occasionally, completely obstructs the flow of blood. As a result, less oxygen flows to affected tissues. The more vital the organ, the more critical this decrease in supply becomes.

Cardiovascular diseases: Diseases of the heart and blood vessels.

Atherosclerosis: Buildup of cholesterol, fat, and cellular debris within the lining of arteries.

Cholesterol A fat-like substance found in animal foods and also manufactured by the body. Cholesterol is essential to nerve and brain cell function and to the synthesis of sex hormones and is also a component of bile acids used to aid fat digestion. It is also a part of atherosclerotic plaques that accumulate on artery walls.

Arteries: Blood vessels carrying oxygenated blood away from the heart toward the tissues.

1

FIGURE 1.1
Atherosclerosis

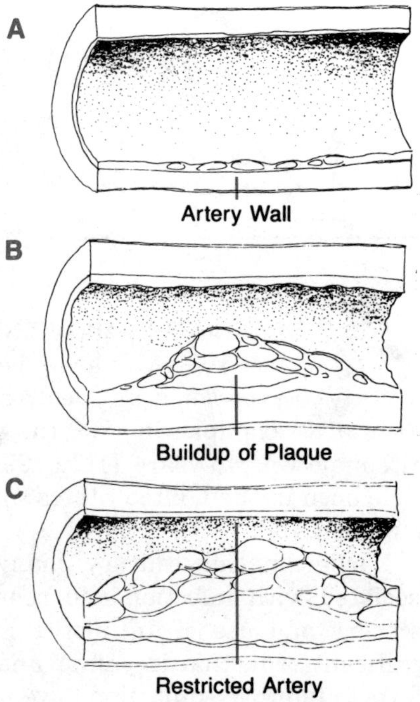

Arteries are the blood vessels that carry oxygenated blood from the heart to the body's tissues and organs.

Atherosclerosis is a buildup of fat, cholesterol, and cellular debris in the inner lining of an artery. This buildup is called plaque and may partially or totally block an artery.

When an artery is partially blocked, less oxygen reaches the affected tissue and damage may occur. If the artery is totally blocked, a heart attack or stroke may result.

A

Artery Wall

B

Buildup of Plaque

C

Restricted Artery

Fatty deposits and their consequence, a hardening of the arteries, occur normally with aging. But poor diet, smoking, and an inactive life-style can speed up the process.

This chapter will review the effects of atherosclerosis on the heart and describe the signs and symptoms of a heart attack. Our discussion will consider each of the major risk factors contributing to heart disease and examine several secondary contributing factors. If you can identify the controllable factors, you can construct a personal plan of action that will decrease your risk of suffering heart disease.

THE CARDIOVASCULAR SYSTEM AT WORK

The heart is primarily a muscle that functions as a pump to supply vital oxygen, carried in the blood, to the body's tissues.

FIGURE 1.2

The Heart at Work

Did You Know That . . .

There are approximately 52,000 miles of blood vessels in the human body.

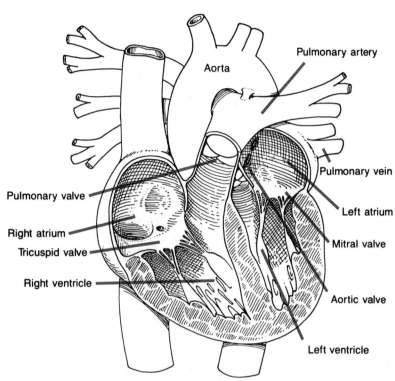

Pulmonary artery

Aorta

Pulmonary vein

Pulmonary valve

Left atrium

Right atrium

Mitral valve

Tricuspid valve

Right ventricle

Aortic valve

Left ventricle

Source: Leonard Dank, Medical Illustrations.

The heart is a powerful muscle that functions as a pump. It is divided into 4 compartments or chambers, a left and right atrium and a left and right ventricle. Freshly oxygenated blood from the lungs enters the left atrium, flows through the mitral valve to the left ventricle, is pumped into the aorta and then to the rest of the body through the arterial system. It returns through the veins to the right atrium, flows through the tricuspid valve into the right ventricle, and is then pumped to the lungs for oxygenation.

About the size of a fist, it lies in the chest behind the sternum (breastbone). The heart has 4 chambers: 2 receive blood (atria) and 2 send blood out (ventricles). One-way valves lie between each chamber to keep the blood flowing in one direction. The valves open and close with each heartbeat, allowing the chambers to fill, then pump.

(continued on p. 5)

Your Heart and How It Works: A Crossword Puzzle

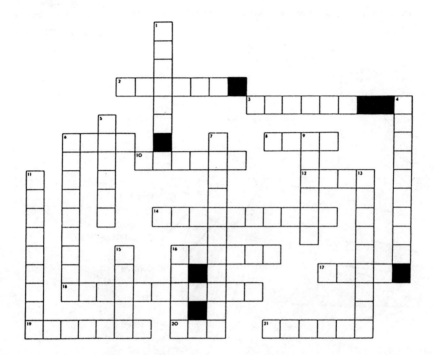

ACROSS:

2. The valve between the left atrium and the left ventricle
3. The heart is classified as a _____
6. Blood vessel which carries blood to the heart
8. The heart is a little larger than your _____
10. _____ regulate the flow of blood through the heart
12. One function of the heart is to _____ blood to the lungs
14. The tough, muscular wall of the heart
16. Upper chamber of the heart
17. From the right side of the heart blood goes to the _____
18. Lining of the heart
19. Waste gas: carbon _____
20. Warning of a heart attack: pain may radiate down the _____
21. Blood vessel which carries blood from the heart

Source: American Heart Association.

DOWN:

1. The valve between the left ventricle and the aorta
4. The valve between the right ventricle and the pulmonary artery
5. The heart pumps blood to each body _____
6. Lower chamber of the heart
7. Fiber-like bag surrounding the heart
9. Wall which divides heart cavity down the middle
11. The valve between the right atrium and the right ventricle
13. The artery/vein connecting lungs and heart
15. _____ is pumped through the body to nourish all of the tissues
16. Great trunk artery that receives blood from the left ventricle

(Answers on page 144)

FIGURE 1.3
The Coronary Arteries

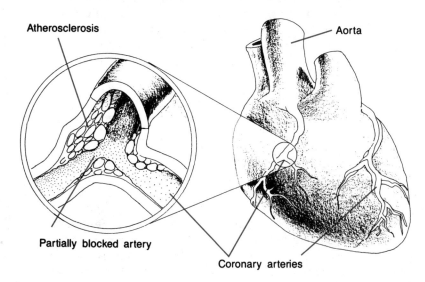

Atherosclerosis

Aorta

Partially blocked artery

Coronary arteries

The heart muscle receives oxygenated blood from the coronary arteries that branch out over the surface of the heart. When plaque builds up inside a portion of a coronary artery, the result may be a heart attack that damages the heart muscle.

Blood exhausted of its oxygen by body tissue travels through blood vessels called **veins**. Venous blood enters the heart in the right **atrium**. It passes through the tricuspid valve into the right **ventricle**. It then travels through the pulmonic valve and out to the lungs through the pulmonary artery. In the lungs, the blood receives new oxygen, releases carbon dioxide (a waste product of metabolism), and returns to the heart's left atrium. This oxygen-rich blood passes through the mitral valve into the left ventricle, the most muscular chamber of the heart. It then travels through the aortic valve into the aorta, the body's largest artery. Arteries carry oxygenated blood away from the heart to all the tissues and organs of the body. After the tissues have taken the oxygen, the blood returns to the heart and the process repeats itself. This cycle occurs with each heartbeat.

The heartbeat is one complete pulsation of the heart that is stimulated by a small mass of tissue, located in the right atrium,

Veins: Blood vessels carrying blood exhausted of its oxygen supply back to the heart.

Atrium: Receiving chamber in the heart.

Ventricle: Pumping chamber in the heart.

Did You Know That . . .

Today, the average person's risk of dying from a heart attack is about 40 percent less than it was for his or her parents at the same age.

Myocardium: Heart muscle.

Coronary arteries: The arteries lying on the surface of the heart muscle that provide the heart with its blood supply.

Ischemia: A chronic reduction in blood supply that results in the inability of the affected organ to function in a normal manner.

Myocardial infarction: The medical term for a heart attack, which means that some of the heart muscle tissue has died.

Arrhythmia: Abnormality of heart rhythm.

that acts as a pacemaker. The pacemaker generates electrical impulses that coordinate the contractions of the atria and the ventricles in a sequential, rhythmic pattern so that blood flows efficiently through the chambers of the heart.

The heart muscle does not get its oxygen and nutrients from the blood that passes through the heart. Rather, these are supplied by blood that reaches the heart muscle, or **myocardium**, from the **coronary arteries**. These arteries, the very first branches off the aorta, lie on the outer surface of the heart.

WHAT IS A HEART ATTACK?

If the blood flow in the coronary arteries diminishes significantly (a condition called **ischemia**), the heart immediately begins to suffer from lack of oxygen. It signals its distress with chest pain. Ischemia is reversible if the artery reopens or if its oxygen demands are reduced, actions that can occur if the heart beats at a lower rate or if blood pressure is reduced to decrease the exertion of the heart. If the blood flow in a coronary artery is entirely blocked, the part of the myocardium that is supplied by the blocked coronary artery may die. If it does, a **myocardial infarction**, or heart attack, has occurred. Most heart attacks result from a blood clot near an area of atherosclerosis that obstructs the flow of blood within the coronary artery. [5] Although one would expect that a person with coronary atherosclerosis should develop symptoms of ischemia prior to having a heart attack, that is not always the case.

An abnormality in the heart's rhythm, called **arrhythmia**, may accompany a heart attack or may merely be a fault of the heart's electrical impulse system. If the abnormal rhythm is associated with a heart attack, it can greatly complicate matters for the victim. Arrhythmia leads to inefficient pumping action and decreases the flow of blood through the arteries even further. If the electrical impulse becomes too chaotic, pumping will cease altogether, resulting in sudden death.

SYMPTOMS OF A HEART ATTACK

Most heart attack patients have one or more warning symptoms. Because early treatment of a heart attack or its warning signs can mean the difference between life and death, it is important to recognize the signs and seek immediate medical attention when

(continued on p. 9)

Heart Attacks: The First Few Minutes

Not only the first few hours after a heart attack but the first few minutes are critical to survival and well-being. Therapy during the first few hours takes place in a hospital; effective treatment in the first few minutes usually must be given at home or on the road.

Dr. John Tobias Nagurney, medical director of the Emergency Department at Cambridge Hospital, Cambridge, Massachusetts, explains what must be done to save heart attack victims before they get to the hospital.

What makes the first few minutes critical?

About one-half of cardiac deaths occur within a couple of hours after the onset of symptoms, and in many of these cases the victim never reaches a hospital. An unexpected collapse, with death in a matter of minutes, is a common scenario. About 80% of sudden deaths result from atherosclerosis; they are heart attacks caused by deficient coronary circulation.

Even though events seem to be moving rapidly to a fatal conclusion, the process leading to sudden death can often be reversed, because it does not come from any intrinsic failure of the heart's strength. Rather, what happens is that the electrical activity coordinating the heart becomes abnormal—there is a sudden life-threatening *arrhythmia*. Instead of pumping blood, the heart just quivers. Unless the circulation can be restored within 4 minutes, the brain is irreversibly damaged and death is the outcome.

If nobody is around when a cardiac arrest takes place, the outcome is almost inevitably fatal. But if the event has witnesses, as is often the case, there is a real hope of saving the person and returning him to life of good quality. (Statistically, men have more heart attacks at younger ages than women do.)

Very occasionally, a hard thump to the chest, delivered by an alert person at the scene, revives someone who has collapsed. The blow evidently triggers a competent portion of the heart to assert its electrical dominance. Although this maneuver is always worth a try, it is rarely successful.

What's the next step?

The next step is to begin cardiopulmonary resuscitation (CPR)—squeezing the heart by rhythmically compressing the chest about once a second and, at intervals of a few seconds, blowing air into the lungs. Mouth-to-mouth breathing is necessary when no equipment is available, although fear of AIDS now deters many people from using this method unless they have specially designed mouthpieces. Rescue teams capable of providing CPR are equipped with so-called ambu bags, which can be used as a mechanical bellows to inflate the lungs. Properly applied, these bags work better than mouth-to-mouth breathing. Maintaining adequate aeration is a crucial element of successful CPR.

The main virtue of CPR is that it can be performed without special equipment and can be initiated immediately after a collapse. If CPR is begun in less than 4 minutes, it appears to make a real contribution to the chances of survival. CPR works better when the people administering it are skilled.

When being performed on a sidewalk, in a bedroom, or in an ambulance, though, CPR has severe limitations. It is not capable of preserving life indefinitely, or even for very long, but it may keep the person going until more effective intervention is possible.

CPR training is available in most communities through local health facilities or the American Red Cross, and I encourage people to enroll in such courses. But it is crucial to recognize that CPR is a stopgap measure. Unless the heart can resume its pumping activity in fairly short order, the outlook is generally not good.

What works better than CPR?

There are some forms of cardiac arrest that don't

respond very well to any intervention. But if the heart has begun to quiver—a condition technically known as *ventricular fibrillation*—there is about a 30–40% chance that appropriate treatment will permit the victim to walk out of the hospital in a week or two. These are optimal statistics, though, derived from communities (such as Seattle, Milwaukee, Oslo, Reykjavik) that have highly organized emergency systems for responding to cardiac arrest.

The intervention that has the best chance of restoring normal electrical activity is to deliver an electric shock across the chest. Known as *defibrillation,* this technique requires putting two paddle-shaped electrodes in a particular position on the chest and delivering a timed current of electricity at an appropriate voltage. The effect of the jolt is to bring the heart to an electrical standstill so that, with luck, one of the heart's natural pacemakers can resume its coordinating activity.

The sooner the heart is defibrillated, the better its owner's chance of recovery. Optimal results require defibrillation in less than 10 minutes and preferably less than 8 minutes from the onset of cardiac arrest. In other words, CPR needs to begin within 4 minutes, and defibrillation in another 4 minutes or so. Seconds count in this situation. A recent study from Seattle compared the elapsed time before CPR was begun and the time before defibrillation was administered in survivors versus nonsurvivors of ventricular fibrillation. In survivors, the average delay until CPR began was 3.6 minutes; it was 6.1 minutes until defibrillation was administered. The corresponding times in nonsurvivors were 4.3 and 7.3 minutes, although there was a good deal of variation in both groups.

This does not mean that CPR should be abandoned after a few minutes. Although the probability of a save goes down, it doesn't disappear. CPR at the scene should continue until a rescue team can arrive and take over.

Defibrillation is easily done in a hospital, but the critical need for it is at a time well before a patient can get to a hospital. So the obvious way to improve a community's response to cardiac emergencies is to put a defibrillating machine in an ambulance and take it to the person who has collapsed—or to the person who has chest pain and shortness of breath and who *might* go into ventricular fibrillation between home and hospital.

How is defibrillation done in the field?

Of course, you can't just send out the machine. You need a crew trained to use it, and the crew has to be able to take an electrocardiogram (EKG) to determine whether ventricular fibrillation really is the problem—because, if it isn't, the shock could do a lot more harm than good. In other words, we're not just talking about a single technological advance that can save lives, but rather about organizing a complex system for delivering "prehospital" care in the form of *advanced life support* (ALS).

Advanced life support systems have been developed over the past 20 years or so. They are well established in many parts of the West and Midwest of the United States but are less widespread in the Northeast. A couple of the best known and most successful programs are in Seattle and Milwaukee. Such programs have reported remarkably high "save rates"—figures as high as 40%, as I mentioned. Without such a system, most communities would have save rates well under 10% and quite possibly in the neighborhood of 1%.

It should be apparent from what I've said that the effectiveness of any system providing emergency care for victims of cardiac arrest depends on rapid response. It's impossible to station a technician at every street corner; so there are two critical factors that depend on the average citizen.

• It may seem trivial, but knowing the telephone number for emergency help is one of the most important. In communities served by the advanced life support system that I work with, people have died during the back-and-forth as a panicked family member called a nearby hospital trying to locate help. The emergency access number is often, but not always, 911; it can be different in adjacent towns.

• Another important element is for a high

percentage of community members to know the very basic techniques of CPR. These may only be helpful if applied within 4 minutes of cardiac arrest, and they may only be good for another 4–5. But those minutes make the difference between life and death.

We had a dramatic example in our own community a couple of years ago. A foreign scholar was attending a university commencement. He collapsed in ventricular fibrillation. A call was placed immediately, CPR was initiated, and, in minutes, an ALS team arrived. He was electrically defibrillated at the scene and taken to the nearest hospital. He was observed there for a few days and then was able to walk out of the building, having suffered no brain damage.

His experience was dramatic but not atypical of people who survive cardiac arrest. In Seattle, a study of people who were alive 6 months after having an out-of-hospital cardiac arrest found that 60% of them were working and the same percentage reported their memory was at least as good as before the arrest; 44% also replied that they could climb stairs as easily as before.

Source: *Harvard Medical School Health Letter,* October 1988, pp. 4–6.

they occur. Pain is the most common symptom. Pain caused by a heart attack usually occurs in the center of the chest. It will often be a dull, aching sensation and may take the form of discomfort or a feeling of tightness, fullness, or squeezing. The discomfort may spread to the jaws, neck, or arms or occur between the shoulder blades. If it lasts more than 2 minutes, take serious measures: Call a doctor. Within 5 minutes, some heart muscle will have started to die. Sweating, nausea, vomiting, dizziness, fainting, anxiety, and/or shortness of breath may accompany the discomfort. The skin may also turn clammy and pale in color. [6]

Because most heart attacks produce only a few of these symptoms, do not wait for more symptoms to occur. Seek medical attention immediately. Time is of the essence.

Did You Know That . . .

Most heart attacks occur between 6:00 A.M. and noon.

HOW TO TELL CHEST PAINS APART

It is not always easy to tell one kind of chest pain from another. If you have occasional or persistent chest pain, it is best to consult your health-care professional for his or her opinion. The following are some guidelines:

1. **Angina pectoris** is the medical term for chest pains that accompany insufficient blood supply to the heart muscle, the physical symptom of ischemia. The ischemia is often reversible with rest. Although angina usually precedes a heart attack, its presence does not mean that a heart attack will invariably occur. As with myocardial infarction, the pain is

Angina pectoris: The medical term for chest pain caused by an insufficient supply of oxygen to the heart muscle.

frequently a dull, aching, squeezing, or smothering discomfort that lies in the center of the chest. Physical activity, emotional stress, cold weather, and especially an activity that requires using your hands over your head may trigger this kind of discomfort. This pain goes away with rest but returns when you resume activity. Activity requires more work from the heart than rest. When you are active, your heart rate and/or blood pressure may rise. This increase in the heart's work load must be matched with an increase in fuel, or oxygen, delivered to the heart. If narrow arteries limit this oxygen delivery, the heart signals its distress with chest discomfort. If you have chest pain that fits this description, see your health-care professional.

2. Chest pains that subside with activity are not likely to be related to the heart. Likewise, sharp, fleeting, "pinprick" sensations are not likely to reflect heart disease. However, some atypical chest pain does imply ischemia. Any unaccountable chest pain is cause for concern and should be called to the attention of your health-care professional.

3. Pain that can be reproduced by pushing on the chest wall is usually due to injury to muscle, bones, or cartilage, and not to heart attack.

4. Heartburn or a stomach ulcer may cause chest pain. This discomfort often occurs when eating or lying down. Antacids may relieve the pain.

WHAT TO DO IF A HEART ATTACK IS OCCURRING

If you are with someone who is having warning signs of an immediate heart attack, action is imperative. Take the following steps as soon as possible:

1. You can expect that the person experiencing chest pain will deny that it is a warning or minimize its seriousness. Don't take "no" for an answer! Act quickly!

2. Dial 911 or call your local emergency rescue/ambulance service immediately. If you can get the victim to a hospital with 24-hour emergency cardiac care in some way that is faster than by waiting for an ambulance, do so.

3. **Cardiopulmonary resuscitation (CPR)** saves lives. CPR involves mouth-to-mouth resuscitation to help restore normal breathing and rhythmic chest compressions, which massage the heart to simulate a heartbeat and maintain the vital blood/oxygen flow through the body. It is given to victims who are not breathing and have no pulse. If you haven't been CPR-trained, do not administer chest compressions. Rather, ask if anyone in your immediate vicinity can administer it until professional help arrives. Most communities offer several sources for CPR instruction to the public.

Arrhythmias are the major cause of deaths that occur during a heart attack. [7] Thirty-five percent of patients who experience an acute myocardial infarction die during the episode. More than half of these die before reaching the hospital. The first few minutes of a heart attack are, therefore, critical. Take warning signs seriously. Have a plan of action for emergencies. Minimize the time it takes for help to arrive. These steps will increase the victim's chances of survival.

DIAGNOSIS AND TREATMENT OF HEART ATTACKS

Usually a physician will make a heart attack diagnosis after reviewing the patient's history as well as the results of his or her physical examination and **electrocardiogram (EKG)**. Sometimes, even with all of that information, a diagnosis is inconclusive. Then blood tests are done every 6 to 8 hours over a 24-hour period to look for a rise in the enzyme creatininephosphokinase (CPK), which is released by dying heart muscle.

Current approaches to treating heart attacks incorporate two strategies. The first is to monitor the patient at all times to detect any abnormal heart rhythms. The second is to minimize the amount of heart muscle destroyed. The second principle is important in preserving the pumping function of the heart. This is achieved by keeping the heart rate and blood pressure normal and by trying to restore blood flow through the affected artery or arteries.

Restoring blood flow through the artery as a method of treatment during a heart attack is a relatively new concept. Two methods became available in the 1980s. The first, **balloon angioplasty**, is a procedure in which a catheter, a very long tube about the size of pencil lead, is introduced through the artery in

Cardiopulmonary resuscitation (CPR) An emergency procedure used to treat someone who is not breathing or whose heart has stopped beating by applying a combination of external cardiac massage and rescue breathing.

Electrocardiogram (EKG): The electrical tracing of the heartbeat.

Balloon angioplasty: Dilating a narrowed artery with a balloon attached to a catheter.

FIGURE 1.4
Balloon Angioplasty

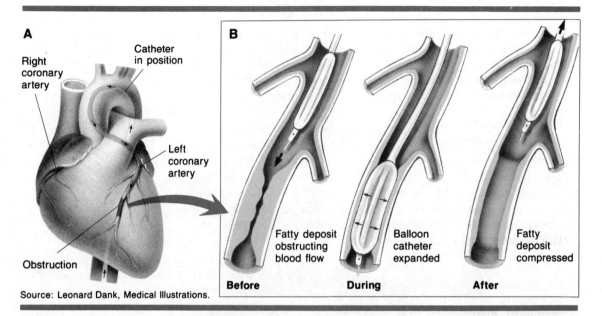

Source: Leonard Dank, Medical Illustrations.

View A shows the heart with an obstructed artery and a balloon catheter in position. View B shows how a balloon is positioned in the artery, inflated, and removed. This procedure compresses the fatty buildup against the artery walls and allows the blood flow to return to near normal.

Lytic drug: Medication used in the treatment of a heart attack that dissolves (or lyses) recently formed blood clots.

Blood clot: A network of blood cells and molecules that solidifies in the bloodstream and stops the flow of blood.

the groin. From there, it travels into the aorta and the coronary artery that has narrowed or been blocked off entirely. The balloon is then inflated to stretch the artery and restore the blood flow so that it is nearly normal. Angioplasty is most effective if used as a preventive device before a heart attack occurs, when angina warns of a problem. The procedure may also be performed 2 to 3 days after a heart attack to prevent further damage.

In these cases, a doctor may want to use a **lytic drug** at the time of the heart attack. Lytic drugs are another method sometimes used to restore blood flow in the coronary arteries. These medications are designed to dissolve any recently developed **blood clot** quickly. The majority of heart attacks are caused by a clot in one of the coronary arteries. If lytic drugs are administered within 2 to 4 hours of the onset of chest pain, they may minimize the amount of heart muscle destroyed in a heart attack. In the case of any heart attack, saving as much muscle as possible is vital.

(continued on p. 15)

Aspirin: Help for the Heart

Almost a century ago, around 1899, an unheralded chemist, working for a German company founded by Friedrich Bayer, developed and patented a drug that eventually landed in millions of medicine cabinets across the world as a remedy to reduce pain and fever. But it was the lowly willow tree that started it all. In the first century A.D. the Greek physician Dioscorides wrote about the medicinal uses of the bark and leaves of the willow; over the centuries, various folk cultures independently discovered that the willow yielded a substance with fever-reducing, pain-killing, anti-inflammatory, and antiseptic properties. The substance was mainly salicin, a cousin of acetasalicylic acid, the active ingredient in aspirin. By the 1830s, researchers had isolated salicin and its derivative, salicylic acid, from the willow. Unfortunately, this version caused too much nausea and stomach discomfort to be widely popular. But the Bayer chemist isolated the salicylic acid without using willow derivatives, making an entirely synthetic drug that had all the therapeutic properties of salicylic acid but with seemingly few side effects, and Bayer aspirin soon became a household name.

Then in the 1960s, researchers discovered that aspirin might have still another—and startling—use: it might prevent heart attacks, the leading cause of death in the United States.

THE CLOT CONNECTION

A myocardial infarction—a heart attack induced by the death of heart muscle—is usually triggered by the formation of a blood clot in the coronary artery. The clot can materialize when a fatty-cholesterol deposit builds up in the artery. The deposit itself is bad enough, because it may narrow the artery, obstructing the flow of blood through it, thereby causing short-duration pains known as angina pectoris. If repeated attacks of sudden severe pain occur, the condition is called unstable angina pectoris and could be a warning sign that clots are forming. The narrowing of the coronary arteries can also cause sudden death

by generating a fatal irregularity (arrhythmia) that makes the heart unable to pump blood anymore. If that weren't enough, a constriction of normal blood flow can also cause coronary spasm, which can either be painful, as in angina, or painless, as in "silent ischemia" (literally, "silent holding back of the blood").

The dismal events caused by fatty-cholesterol deposits and blood clots are not restricted to the heart; they can take place in arteries anywhere in the body. For instance, a stroke may occur if a clot blocks blood flow to a part of the brain. A different, but less common, type of stroke—a hemorrhagic stroke—strikes when an artery in the brain breaks.

ASPIRIN AND HEART HEALTH

Aspirin can do nothing to prevent fatty-cholesterol buildup in the arteries. Nor can it forestall a hemorrhagic stroke (and may, as we'll see, even be risky here). But it can apparently be highly effective in preventing heart attacks and strokes caused by blood clots. And it is clots that account for 85% of all heart attacks, brought on by interruption of blood flow and subsequent death of heart muscle.

Aspirin works its magic by acting as a "blood-thinner." It blocks the normal production of certain prostaglandins (hormone-like substances produced by cells throughout the body), one of which, thromboxane, prompts the platelet substances in the blood to clump together, causing clots. And even tiny doses of aspirin seem to stymie the formation of thromboxane, thereby reducing the blood's ability to clot.

The use of aspirin as a heart helper came about when researchers found that aspirin could reduce the risk of subsequent heart attacks in survivors of a first one and in persons who had a myocardial infarction in progress, had unstable angina pectoris, or had already had a stroke. The intriguing question then was, could aspirin be used to forestall a first heart attack? The answer was a definite yes.

The heartening conclusion was based on a striking study reported in the July 20, 1989, issue of the *New England Journal of Medicine.* The study of 22,071 male physicians over a 5-year period revealed that those who took aspirin were only half as likely to suffer a heart attack as those who didn't. Of course, the results of such a study cannot be applied across the board, because it pertained only to men, and to unusually healthy men at that, who therefore were hardly representative of the general population. Nevertheless, the results still hold water, because the researchers divided the men into two completely comparable groups. Half the men took 325 mg of aspirin every other day; the other half did not. The upshot: there were 139 myocardial infarctions (and 10 deaths) in the aspirin-taking group, but 239 (and 28 deaths) in the aspirin-abstaining group.

Another finding was, however, that aspirin did not prevent sudden deaths, there being only 12 sudden deaths in the nonaspirin group, but 22 in the aspirin group. Sudden deaths, though, are frequently associated not with a clot but with a fatal cardiac irregularity, which is usually caused by fatty-cholesterol deposits in the arteries (and, as we've noted, aspirin can't prevent that plaque buildup).

All of which means that we can't rely on aspirin alone to prevent death from coronary artery disease but should try to prevent those unseemly deposits by keeping our total cholesterol and blood pressure sufficiently low.

DOES ASPIRIN AFFECT THE RISK FACTORS?

Advancing age, high cholesterol levels, high blood pressure, smoking, alcohol, and physical inactivity are regarded as likely to predispose a person to the development of heart disease. Does taking aspirin make these risk factors less risky?

Aging. It was in the men 50 years of age or older that aspirin was most effective in preventing a heart attack. Those 50 to 84 years old who took aspirin had only about half as many heart attacks as those who, in all age groups over 50, didn't.

High cholesterol levels. Of the men whose total cholesterol level was 210 mg/dl or higher, the aspirin group had only about 60% as many heart attacks as did the nonaspirin group. Even when the total cholesterol level was below 210, the aspirin users had only a third as many heart attacks as did the nonusers.

High blood pressure. Aspirin apparently did not decrease the risk posed by high blood pressure.

Alcohol. Whether the men took aspirin or not, the risk caused by alcohol remained just about the same. (Interestingly, whether the men drank alcohol daily, weekly, or rarely, the alcohol did not protect the heart from an attack—a finding that puts in question the widely held belief that alcohol protects the heart.) In any case, combining aspirin with alcohol can cause irritation, and even bleeding, of the stomach.

Smoking. The use of cigarettes seemed to have no bearing on aspirin's beneficial effect. Whether the men were currently smokers, were past smokers, or had never smoked, aspirin still cut their risk of a myocardial infarction by more than 50%. But this finding should hardly encourage smokers to breathe (if they can) a sigh of relief: as aspirin cannot cancel the risk caused by use of the weed, smoking remains a potential killer.

Physical inactivity. Although aspirin appeared to be just about as effective in men who exercised regularly and vigorously as in the few men who were sluggards, there was an interesting bit of difference: aspirin gave more protection to the nonexercisers. The possible explanation: Exercise may have already initiated an anti-clotting effect by stimulating the release of TPA (tissue plasminogen activator), a protein with a potent ability to dissolve clots. So the exercisers had the jump on the nonexercisers, who relied on aspirin alone to keep their blood unclotted.

THE STROKE STORY

When aspirin was used by survivors of a stroke caused by a blood clot, it reduced the risk of a second stroke. But among the aspirin takers there were 119 strokes, and among the aspirin abstainers 98—not really much difference with such relatively small numbers. And although there were 23 *hemorrhagic* strokes in the aspirin groups and only 12 in the nonaspirin one, the comparatively few strokes of this type suggest that the risk is rather small. Imbibing even moderate amounts of alcohol seems to increase the risk of a hemorrhagic stroke far more than taking aspirin does.

SOME DANGERS OF ASPIRIN USE

Gastrointestinal discomfort, one of the well-known side effects of aspirin use, was reported by 26.1% of the aspirin takers, but it was also a complaint of 25.6% of those who didn't take any aspirin, so the difference was negligible. The former group did have more ulcers (169) than the latter (138), but the total number of ulcers was small—less than 1.4% among more than 22,000 men. But because aspirin inhibits blood clotting, 38 of the aspirin users had bleeding ulcers, whereas only 22 of the nonusers did. Other hemorrhagic problems also were more prevalent among the aspirin takers: 2,979 of them (731 more than the nonusers) vomited blood, passed blood in the stool, bruised more easily, and had nosebleeds.

Clearly, aspirin use is not recommended for anyone who already has a bleeding ulcer, is taking blood-thinning medication, or has recently had surgery.

CONCLUSIONS

For men over 50 (and possibly women, too, but that still has to be ironed out), taking 325 mg of aspirin every other day may well decrease their risk of a first heart attack—that is, myocardial infarction—and, possibly, premature death. Although aspirin does not seem able to defend against sometimes lethal heart disorders unrelated to blood clots, nor against a first stroke (and may even help precipitate a hemorrhagic one), its use in guarding the heart still seems justified.

Remember, though, that aspirin merely decreases the risk of a heart attack—it doesn't *eliminate* that risk. So we can't depend on it to do all the work. We still have to fight artery disease by reducing fat intake, lowering high blood pressure and high cholesterol levels, drinking prudently if at all, exercising, and not smoking.

Because aspirin inhibits blood clotting for at least 48 hours, only one 325 mg tablet every other day is needed. If you're not sure about the state of your heart (medically speaking, that is) and are thinking about taking aspirin over a long period, be sure to consult with your physician first. And then, with all due respect to the apple, perhaps you can start saying, "An aspirin every other day keeps the doctor away."

—Lieselotte Hofmann

Source: *Healthline,* February 1990, pp. 8–10.

Once a blood clot has been dissolved, medications that inhibit the clotting of the blood are often used with heart attack victims. Aspirin, for example, has some anti-clotting effects that have been shown to help prevent heart attacks or their recurrence. [8] Aspirin acts by making platelets (blood cells necessary in the clotting process) less capable of adhering to each other and to the blood vessels, so that blood clots are less likely to form.

Nitroglycerin is another medication that has long been used with heart patients. Its primary action is to dilate blood vessels, arteries, or veins. Often used intravenously at the time of a heart attack, nitroglycerin in pill form can be used to help abate the pain of angina.

Thanks to more advanced medical treatment of heart attack patients, about 80 percent of people who survive a heart attack are now able to return to work and other normal activities within 3 months.

FIGURE 1.5
Coronary Bypass Surgery

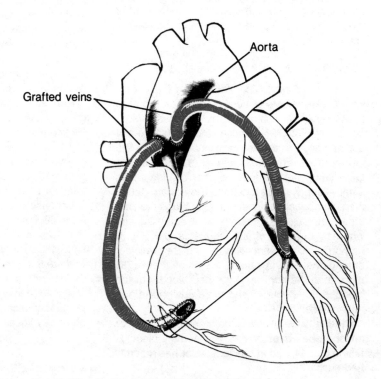

Source: *Understanding Angina*, American Heart Association, p. 8.

During coronary bypass surgery, a vein from the leg is used to bypass the blockage in the coronary artery or arteries.

Medications to help regulate heart rhythm can also help people experiencing a heart attack. Lidocaine is used most frequently for this purpose. It is also often used to help prevent a life-threatening arrhythmia, especially within the first 24 hours. [9] Digitalis derivatives also help regulate the heart's rhythm and over a long period of time may actually strengthen contractions of the heart muscle.

Finally, bypass surgery is a form of treatment for narrowed or obstructed arteries. However, this procedure is rarely done at

the time of a heart attack. Instead, it is performed when progressive chest discomfort means a heart attack is likely. Surgeons
performing bypass procedures redirect blood around the narrowed portion of the coronary artery and back to the heart
muscle. This is done by grafting an artery or vein that has been
removed from elsewhere in the patient's body onto the affected
coronary artery. Double, triple, and quadruple bypasses refer to
the number of arteries bypassed.

PREVENTING HEART ATTACKS

Unfortunately, the first symptom of atherosclerosis may be the
last, namely, a heart attack or **stroke**. Preventing or minimizing
the effects of atherosclerosis is easier than suffering a heart
attack. The good news is that atherosclerosis can be prevented or
its progression slowed. By lowering our cholesterol levels and
quitting smoking while at the same time controlling other risk
factors, we can prevent, reverse, or slow the progress of atherosclerosis. [10]

Major Risk Factors
Scientists don't know the specific way in which atherosclerosis
develops. However, they have studied many of the risk factors
that contribute to its development. Most of these major risk
factors can be eliminated or minimized by making changes in our
life-style.
    Consider cigarette smoking. The risk of developing and
dying from coronary heart disease is 3 to 5 times higher in
smokers than in nonsmokers. The risk increases with the number
of cigarettes smoked per day. For reasons as yet unknown, statistics show that a heart attack in a smoker is more likely to be fatal
than a heart attack in a nonsmoker. Sudden death as the first
symptom of heart disease is 2 to 3 times more likely to occur in
35- to 54-year-old male cigarette smokers than in nonsmokers.
And smoking when combined with other risk factors multiplies
the effect of all the risk factors. That smoking affects arteries is
well established. However, the mechanism by which such changes
occur is not yet known. Evidence suggests that nicotine, carbon
monoxide, and arterial narrowing each play a role.
    The increased risk of heart disease that cigarette smoking
causes is reversible, though, if the smoker quits his or her habit.
For example, 1 year after quitting, risk of heart disease lessens by
25 percent. Ten years after stopping, a person with a pack-a-day

Stroke: Damage to part of the
brain caused by interruption
to its blood supply, resulting
in physical or mental
impairment or even death.

habit reduces his or her risk of heart disease to the same level as someone who has never smoked. The message here is, don't start smoking, or if you do smoke, stop.

You can stop smoking abruptly and completely (known as "cold turkey") without physical harm. [11] In such instances, it may be helpful to substitute another behavior—chewing gum, for example—during the times that you usually smoked. Prescription nicotine gum is available if you are addicted to nicotine. "Stop Smoking" clinics and support groups have been successful in helping some eliminate the habit. You will find more discussion about stopping smoking in chapter 6.

Another major risk factor is high blood pressure. Also referred to as hypertension, high blood pressure causes the heart to work harder. It also doubles the risk of developing atherosclerotic heart disease. When high blood pressure is combined with smoking and elevated cholesterol levels, a multiplying effect occurs. In other words, the presence of 3 risk factors produces a likelihood of developing heart disease that is 10 times greater than the likelihood of heart disease in someone without any risk factors.

Since high blood pressure is usually without symptoms, it is known as the "silent disease." The only way to detect its presence is to have periodic blood pressure checks, a simple and painless procedure. The 1988 Report of the Joint National Committee on Detection, Evaluation and Treatment of High Blood Pressure recommends a blood pressure screening every 2 years for individuals with a blood pressure under 140/90. [12] Those with blood pressure measurements above 140/90 should be checked within 2 months to verify the elevated reading because they are at a higher risk of suffering heart disease. A person having 3 separate resting blood pressure readings greater than 140/90 should be treated with medication.

The cause of high blood pressure is not yet known. In affluent societies, blood pressure increases with age. According to several studies, blacks in the United States have a greater chance of having elevated blood pressure than whites. [13] A family history of high blood pressure also increases an individual's risk. Obesity and excessive salt intake may increase the risk as well. Treatment may consist of weight loss, exercise, restricted salt intake, and medication.

A third risk factor is elevated cholesterol. There is significant evidence to correlate a high fat diet with premature coronary artery disease. Finland's diet is highest in fat, and, even though the Finns are more active than Americans overall, they have the world's highest rate of heart disease. Scotland, Northern

FIGURE 1.6
Coronary Heart Disease Rates in Seven Countries

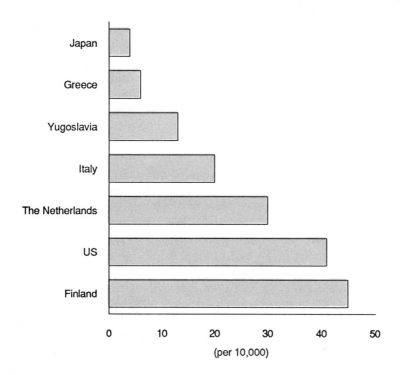

(per 10,000)

Source: A. Keys, *Seven Countries: A Multivariate Analysis of Death and Coronary Heart Disease* (Cambridge, MA: Harvard University Press, 1980).

This chart shows that in the countries studied, Finland has the highest death rate from heart disease. There is significant evidence to correlate the high-fat diet of the Finnish people with the high rate of heart disease.

Ireland, Australia, New Zealand, England, and the United States aren't far behind Finland. The lowest cholesterol levels and the lowest death rates from atherosclerosis come from the Latin American countries and Japan. [14] However, studies have shown that people who move to the United States from one of the countries with a lower incidence of heart disease develop a higher risk of suffering heart disease than their relatives of the same age who remain at home. [15]

Did You Know That . . .

Despite the accumulation of evidence that tobacco use is a major risk factor for coronary heart disease, the number of women who smoke has declined only 16 percent since 1965, while the number of men who smoke has dropped by 36 percent.

A person's cholesterol level is determined by age, sex, heredity, and diet. [16] The first 3 factors are unchangeable. Diet, which is very important, is determined by the individual. A low-fat, low-cholesterol diet does decrease a person's cholesterol level. Lowering the cholesterol level decreases the risk of coronary heart disease. [17]

An elevated cholesterol level is defined as a blood cholesterol level greater than 240 mg/dl (milligrams/deciliter). A blood cholesterol measure between 200 and 239 mg/dl is considered borderline. A cholesterol level less than 200 mg/dl in middle-aged adults seems to indicate a relatively lower risk of coronary heart disease. Blood cholesterol levels should be checked beginning at age 20. Those with normal levels should be tested every 5 years. More frequent checks are in order for those with borderline or elevated cholesterol levels. [18]

Elevated blood cholesterol is also called **hyperlipidemia**. A more complete description occurs in chapter 5, along with dietary recommendations to lower blood cholesterol levels.

Reversible Diabetes Risk Factors
A final major risk factor is **diabetes**. Adult-onset diabetes (affecting about 75 percent of diabetics) is inherited and occurs primarily in people over 35 years of age who are overweight and inactive. Diabetics have more coronary heart disease and more heart attacks than people without diabetes. Diabetes increases the damage to blood vessels of its victims by accelerating the process of atherosclerosis. Diabetes, high blood pressure, and an elevated cholesterol level in combination significantly increase the risk of heart disease.

A well-balanced, low-fat, calorie-specific diet, along with exercise, is essential to controlling diabetes and decreasing the harm it does to blood vessels. Medications are sometimes needed as well. Treatment is important not only to control the diabetes but to decrease the risk of coronary artery disease.

Other Risk Factors
Other risk factors play a role in the development of premature coronary artery disease. These include obesity, inactivity, stress, and the use of oral contraceptives. Although independently they are not risk factors, together they can become so and can influence the development of heart disease.

Obesity   There are two distinct, genetically determined patterns of weight gain. The male type is described as apple-shaped—a large

Hyperlipidemia: Elevated levels of fats in the blood.

Diabetes: A disorder characterized by abnormally high levels of glucose (sugar) in the blood resulting from the failure of the pancreas to produce a sufficient supply of insulin, the hormone responsible for the conversion of glucose into a form usable by the cells of the body.

FIGURE 1.7
The Health Benefits of Exercise

Benefits for your heart: Aerobic exercise raises the heart rate to a predetermined "target level" and maintains that level for at least 15 to 20 minutes. This increases the size and stamina of the heart muscle, resulting in a lower resting heart rate. Aerobic exercise also improves the efficiency of the heart, allowing it to pump a greater volume of blood with each beat. One result is a reduced risk of heart disease and heart attack.

Benefits for your circulation: Exercise increases the amount of oxygen in the bloodstream, and the level of HDL cholesterol in the blood, which reduces the level of harmful fats. It lowers blood pressure thus helping to prevent stroke and heart attack. It stimulates the growth of new blood vessels which improve the distribution of oxygenated blood to the body and provide a possible alternate route to organs whose blood supply might otherwise be cut off by blocked passageways.

Benefits for your muscles: Exercise increases the supply of oxygen to muscles while strengthening and toning them. It may also improve coordination.

Benefits for your joints: Exercise keeps the joints supple and prevents joint disorders by strengthening the cartilage.

Benefits for your bones: Exercise thickens the bones and inhibits the loss of calcium associated with osteoporosis.

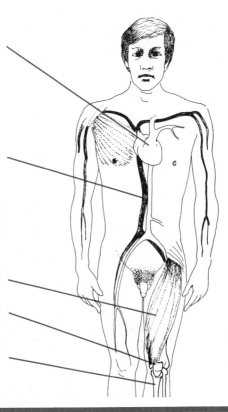

Besides tightening and toning muscles, aerobic exercise also strengthens the heart, stimulates the building of new blood vessels which promotes better circulation, and often reduces the level of fat in the blood.

4. Avoid "energy savers," such as remote-control TV channel changers and golf carts.

5. Walk, don't drive, on errands that are within a mile (20 minutes walking time) of your home.

Stress It is generally accepted that emotional stress may trigger an episode of angina. Blood pressure and heart rate do rise with emotional stress. In addition, it has been suggested that abdomen and small hips. The female type is pear-shaped—a small waist and large hips. While male-pattern obesity predominates in men, it may occur in either men or women. Similarly, female-pattern obesity does not occur exclusively in women. So-called apple-shaped obesity is strongly associated with elevated cholesterol, high blood pressure, and elevated blood sugar. [19] Pear-shaped obesity has a much lower association with these risk factors. Obesity, then, is more significant for those with male-pattern obesity. They are the ones most likely to benefit from weight loss. Losing weight through exercise and a sensible diet lowers the risk for coronary heart disease by reducing the cholesterol level, blood pressure, and risk of diabetes.

Physical Inactivity Lack of exercise has recently been established as a risk factor for heart disease. The U.S. government's *1990 Objectives for the Nation,* for example, set as a goal that 60 percent of those between ages 18 and 65 participate in levels of physical activity sufficient for cardiorespiratory benefit. Current exercise patterns in Americans fall far short of that goal. [20] Regular, vigorous, and life-long physical activity does protect against heart attack risk. Physical inactivity, on the other hand, often combined with overeating, leads to another risk factor, obesity. [21]

There are many benefits of exercise. A vigorous and physically active life-style frequently encourages an interest in good nutrition and discourages such unhealthful habits as cigarette smoking. With regular, **aerobic exercise**, diabetics may decrease their need for medication and may improve blood sugar levels. Choose physical activities that can be continued for a lifetime. There are many types of aerobic exercise from which to choose, including regular brisk walking, jogging, running, dancing, swimming, skiing, and bicycling.

In addition to incorporating regular aerobic exercise 3 times a week, 15 to 30 minutes each time, you may want to burn off calories through other small changes in your life-style. While specific exercise guidelines appear in chapter 6, here are some helpful preliminary suggestions:

1. Walk or bicycle all or partway to work or school.

2. Use stairs rather than elevators.

3. Develop hobbies, such as gardening and other outdoor pursuits, that require physical activity.

Did You Know That . .

Walking a mile in 12 utes burns the : number of calories as jogg mile in 8 and one-half min

Aerobic exercise: A form of exercise that increases respiration, intake of oxygen, heart rate, and cardiovascular fitness.

those who suffer severe emotional stress or have a **Type A** personality have an increased risk of developing heart disease. Considerable public attention has been focused on Type A behavior, which is said to include excessive smoking, poor eating habits, and a preoccupation with time. However, it is not known whether one's personality type may actually make heart disease more likely. [22]

By itself, stress does not cause heart disease. However, someone with heart disease may have to learn new ways to cope with stress or to avoid stressful situations. People in whom heart disease and maladaptive behavior are combined may need counseling or additional medical treatment. Adequate sleep, good nutritional habits, and exercise are among the steps recommended to help relieve stress that are easiest to implement.

Oral Contraceptives   Oral contraceptives, or birth control pills, are an effective way for women to prevent pregnancy. They are convenient and, for most women, free of serious side effects. Most oral contraceptives have a combination of **estrogen** and **progesterone**, the two female hormones, and work principally by preventing the release of an egg from the ovary. In general, increased amounts of estrogen in a pill increase the chance of serious side effects on the woman taking it. Serious side effects include a blood clot, a heart attack, or a stroke. As a result of these findings, most oral contraceptives today have a very low estrogen content (35 micrograms each or less) to minimize the risk of serious side effects.

Blood clots are the most common of the serious side effects of oral contraceptives. A blood clot can cause a heart attack if it forms in a coronary artery. It can cause a stroke if it forms in an artery supplying the brain. A clot can form in the legs or pelvis, break off, and travel to the lungs to cause a **pulmonary embolism**. Each of these events—a heart attack, stroke, or pulmonary embolism—may cause death. These problems occur more frequently in women who use oral contraceptives and are over 40, or in women who use oral contraceptives, are over 35, and smoke.

This discussion of the possible serious side effects of the birth control pill must be put into perspective. Death rates for women aged 13 to 35 are lower for women who use the pill than for women who use no form of contraception. That is because of the death rate associated with pregnancy. [23] Furthermore, the serious side effects of the pill are rare. If you use oral contraceptives, make sure your health-care practitioner is monitoring your health. Discuss any concerns you have about significant adverse

(continued on p. 25)

Type A: A pattern of behavior characterized by overwork, hostility, inability to relax, and a tendency to hurry.

Estrogen: A female sex hormone responsible for secondary sex characteristics and for providing a suitable environment for conception during the menstrual cycle.

Progesterone: A female sex hormone that plays a major role in the menstrual cycle.

Pulmonary embolism: A blood clot that travels to the lung.

Women and Heart Disease: An Equal Opportunity

**Danger of Heart Attack
by Risk Factors Present**
Example: 55-year-old male and female

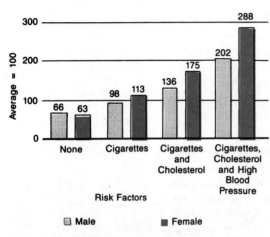

Risk Factors

☐ Male   ■ Female

This chart shows how a combination of three major risk factors can increase the likelihood of heart attack. For purposes of illustration, this chart uses an abnormal blood pressure level of 150 systolic and a cholesterol level of 260 in a 55-year-old male and female.

Source: Framingham Heart Study, Section 37: The Probability of Developing Certain Cardiovascular Diseases in Eight Years at Specified Values of Some Characteristics (August 1987).

As the chart above shows, an average 55-year-old American woman has about the same danger of heart attack as an average 55-year-old man—and her risk is even greater than his if it is compounded by risk factors. In fact, the average American woman can expect to live a third of her life at high risk for heart disease, says Dr. Barbara Packard of the National Heart, Lung and Blood Institute, and a member of the American Heart Association's (AHA) Women and Heart Disease Task Force. One in nine women between the ages of 45 and 64 already has coronary heart disease (CHD), as does one in three of those over 65. It's far more probable that a woman, like a man, will die of CHD than of anything else: As opposed to a one in 10 chance of dying of breast

cancer, for example, a woman's risk of dying of CHD is one in two.

Despite these ominous figures, CHD has traditionally been positioned as a "man's disease"—and research dollars have focused on taking care of men. The result of this misconception and misspending is that too few women take their heart health seriously enough. And too few doctors take the heart health of their female patients seriously enough—or if they do, they don't know how to help. So while deaths from CHD in this country have dropped precipitously over the past 15 years, the decline for women has been far less impressive than that for men.

One reason that the research spotlight has been on men is because they are younger, often in their forties, when they start showing evidence of CHD. Women tend to develop heart disease later in life, usually after menopause. Older age makes them more prone to complications if they undergo bypass surgery or angioplasty. But if they are aware that heart disease might be brewing, women can turn this time lag to their advantage and use it as a 10-year buffer zone to catch up on the same heart-healthy habits that have helped men. Late last year, the AHA launched a major initiative to alert women to the need to pay attention to the health of their heart. The emphasis is on preventing CHD by cutting risk factors and having regular checkups that include monitoring to facilitate early detection.

The best medicine
Since women get CHD later in life, when it can be harder to treat, preventing the process in the first place may be even more important for them than it is for men. The benchmark Framingham Heart Study showed that women have the same risk factors for heart disease as men. The mechanism by which these factors lead to heart disease in women seems to be somewhat different than it is in men—but advice on how women can reduce their risks is, by and large, grounded in studies on men. For example, doctors are quick to advise

men to keep their cholesterol levels below 200 milligrams per deciliter; such a baseline hasn't been definitively set for women because of a dearth of studies.

Research dollars have been belatedly earmarked to determine accurate goals for women to strive for, and several large-scale studies are now under way. For example, one recent study reported in the *New England Journal of Medicine* found that women who quit smoking cut their risk of a first heart attack to nearly that of a non-smoker in just three years. The safest course for now is for women to control lifestyle risks just as much as men, and in the same ways.

Early detection

There's a bias in how doctors monitor women for CHD. In one study, 13 male internists viewed videotapes of two actors portraying patients complaining of heart pain. Both were supposedly smokers who had stressful jobs—but one was male and the other female. Two-thirds of the doctors recommended that the man undergo further evaluation; only a third suggested the same for the woman. Even more shocking—all 13 doctors recommended that the man stop smoking; *none* made such a recommendation to the woman. Two doctors did recommend that the woman see a psychiatrist, however.

It's a tall order, but the way for women to circumvent such discrimination is to be more active participants in their health care. "Women have got to self-screen themselves for heart disease risk, and they've got to push their doctors to pay attention to them," says Dr. Myron Weisfeldt, president of the AHA and a Johns Hopkins cardiologist. Experts say that the presence of CHD can be accurately detected in over 90% of women, using a combination of noninvasive tests. The most common of these are the exercise stress test (which uses an electrical tracing—an EKG—to monitor heart function at different levels of exertion) and the more exacting nuclear imaging exercise stress test (which monitors blood flow to the heart at different levels of exertion with a scanner that traces the progress of a radioactive dye into the heart; the dye is administered prior to the test).

But you have to make sure your doctor refers you for such evaluative tests if you are at risk. Tell your doctor that you want to be closely monitored for CHD if you have any of the risk factors [outlined on page 26]. If he or she dismisses your concerns, find another doctor. Also, ask your doctor for a frank discussion of the pros and cons of hormone therapy, based on your risk factors. (Note: Your gynecologist should not be treating your heart. You should be evaluated and monitored by an internist.)

You must also be aware of angina, the cardinal symptom of CHD: chest pain that starts when you exercise or exert yourself and is relieved by rest. Any unusual chest pain that persists despite rest should send you directly to the emergency room.

Source: *Johns Hopkins Medical Letter, Health After 50,* August 1990, pp. 4–5.

effects of the pill with him or her. If you are on the pill and smoke, you need to stop smoking.

Major Unchangeable Risk Factors: Age, Gender, Heredity

Some risk factors associated with heart disease cannot be changed. These include:

1. *Age:* Increasing age is a risk factor for developing coronary heart disease. However, this alone is not an overwhelming

(continued on p. 27)

Unchangeable risk factors:

- **Genetics.** If you have a parent or sibling who died of premature CHD (before age 65), your risk increases.
- **Race.** Until age 74, black women are twice as likely to die of CHD as white women; after age 75, white women are more likely to die of CHD.

Evaluating Your Risk for Coronary Heart Disease

- **Age.** Risk of CHD increases with age. Nearly 55% of all heart attack victims are 65 or older. At older ages, women who have heart attacks are twice as likely as men to die from them within a few weeks.

Controllable risk factors:

- **Smoking.** For women, smoking is the most significant risk factor for heart disease. If you smoke, you more than double your risk of having a heart attack. And your chances of dying from it—and of dying suddenly, within an hour—are also greater. However, your heart disease risk rapidly declines if you stop smoking, no matter how long or how much you've smoked.
- **High blood pressure.** More than half of all women 55 and over have hypertension (blood pressure of 140/90 or above) and the rate is even higher for black women. Women 65 and older are more likely to develop hypertension than men.
- **Elevated cholesterol.** If your cholesterol level is high—over 240 milligrams per deciliter (mg/dl)—you have twice the risk of developing CHD than at levels below 200 mg/dl. Your risk may also be elevated if your HDL ("good" cholesterol) level is low.
- **Obesity.** Your risk of heart disease increases if you are more than 30% over your ideal weight, even if you have no other risk factor. New research suggests that this risk may be elevated even if you are closer to your ideal weight.
- **Physical inactivity.** Many studies have shown an association between inactivity and heart disease. Inactivity often goes hand in hand with obesity, another risk factor.
- **Stress.** The relationship between CHD and a stressful life also seems to be secondary. Women who feel stressed appear to be more likely to smoke, for example, or have other lifestyle habits that are unhealthy for the heart.
- **Diabetes.** More than 80% of people with diabetes die of some form of heart or blood vessel disease. Women with diabetes have twice the risk of developing CHD as nondiabetic women.

Source: "Women and Heart Disease: An Equal Opportunity," *Johns Hopkins Medical Letter; Health After 50,* August 1990, p. 5.

factor. There are 60-year-old people with coronary arteries as healthy as a 20-year-old's.

2. *Gender:* Coronary heart disease develops 10 to 15 years later in women than in men. Typically, males may exhibit symptoms of heart disease in their 60s while females may not have symptoms until in their 70s.

3. *Heredity:* The tendency of members of some families to have heart attacks and atherosclerosis at an early age can be attributed to hereditary factors. Elevated cholesterol levels, too, can be attributed to genetic traits. However, people with elevated cholesterol levels that result from heredity can be helped by a cholesterol-lowering life-style and a proper diet.

In fact, you need not despair if any of these unchangeable risk factors seems to put you at a disadvantage in preventing heart disease. Obviously, you can't change your age, sex, race, or genetic inheritance. However, there is general agreement that increased cholesterol levels, high blood pressure, and cigarette smoking may be the most important risk factors involved in developing atherosclerosis. [24] And those are risk factors that are under our control. ⟨W⟩

CHAPTER

2

Other Cardiovascular Diseases

DISEASES OF THE HEART and blood vessels remain the number-one killers in the United States. Understanding these diseases is paramount to their prevention, and for those that aren't preventable, we can minimize their effects. This chapter addresses the problems of high blood pressure, stroke, and other forms of heart disease. It also offers suggestions on ways to deal with the problems should they arise and a plan to help prevent them.

HIGH BLOOD PRESSURE

Fifty-eight million Americans—nearly 25 percent of the population—have high blood pressure. Older people in particular are susceptible; 52 percent of women and 44 percent of men over 65 years of age suffer the condition. In addition to age, obesity and a sedentary life-style increase the likelihood of high blood pressure. Other risk factors include race, heredity, and gender. [1]

What Is Blood Pressure?
As blood travels through arteries, it pushes against the arterial walls. This force against the arteries' walls is called blood pressure.

Arteries are muscular and elastic so that they stretch and contract when pumped blood courses through them. Each heartbeat consists of a **systolic** and a **diastolic** phase. The systolic phase occurs when the heart pumps blood out to the body. The diastolic, or resting phase, occurs when the heart fills with blood returning through the veins. Blood pressure is an expression of the burden of the pumping action on your heart and arteries. A

Systolic: The pumping phase of the heartbeat, reflected in the first or higher number of the blood pressure reading.

Diastolic: The filling phase of the heartbeat, reflected in the second or lower number of the blood pressure reading.

FIGURE 2.1

Estimated Percent of Population with Hypertension by Race and Sex, U.S. Adults Age 18–74

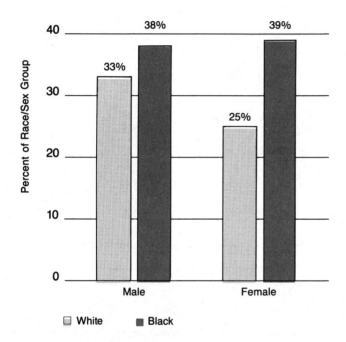

Hypertensives are defined as persons with a systolic level > 140 and/or a diastolic level > 90 or who report using antihypertensive medication.

Source: American Heart Association, *1991 Heart and Stroke Facts,* p. 12.

As the above figure indicates, the incidence of hypertension is greater among white males than among white females and is generally greater among blacks than whites.

typical blood pressure for a healthy young person is 120/80. When the pumping heart produces maximum pressure against the arteries, the measurement for the systolic blood pressure is taken, represented by the first and higher of the two numbers. The lower number, which registers when the heart is filling, is the diastolic blood pressure. The higher the numbers, the greater the burden on the heart.

Did You Know That . . .

A bout 7 percent of all people age 60 to 69 develop what is called isolated hypertension, a condition in which the systolic blood pressure can rise suddenly to 160 millimeters of mercury (mm Hg) or more, but the diastolic pressure remains at the normal value of less than 90 mm Hg.

FIGURE 2.2
Systolic and Diastolic Phases of the Heartbeat

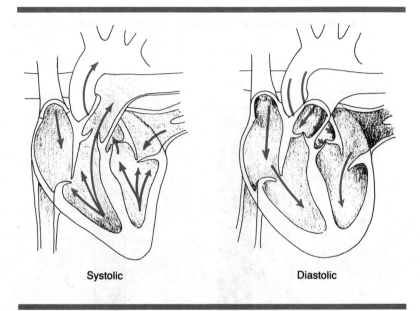

Systolic   Diastolic

During the systolic phase the heart muscle contracts and blood is pumped out of the heart. The diastolic phase occurs when the heart muscle relaxes and fills with blood.

Taking one's blood pressure reading requires a blood pressure cuff and a stethoscope. The cuff is wrapped around the upper arm and inflated with air until it stops the flow of blood through the arteries. As the air in the cuff is slowly released, the flow through the arteries returns. When the arterial pressure exceeds the cuff pressure, the pulse will be heard with the stethoscope. The first time the pulse is heard is the systolic blood pressure. The diastolic blood pressure is noted when the pulse is no longer heard.

Although there is no ideal blood pressure, lower blood pressure lessens one's atherosclerotic risk. Acceptable blood pressures fall within a limited range. For most adults, a blood pressure reading up to 140/90 is acceptable.

What Is High Blood Pressure?
Arterioles, small vessels that have branched off from the arteries, regulate blood pressure. Arterioles work like the nozzle on

FIGURE 2.3
Blood Pressure Test

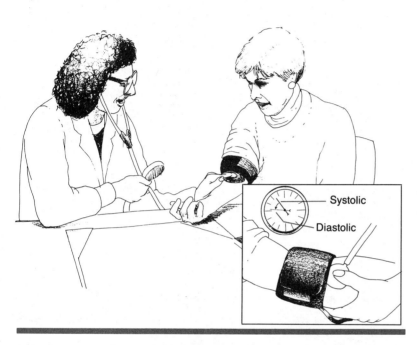

Systolic

Diastolic

A blood pressure cuff and stethoscope are used to measure blood pressure. The cuff is inflated to stop the flow of blood. When it is gradually deflated, blood begins to force its way through the arteries in the arm. The reading taken the first time the pulse can be heard is the systolic blood pressure. The diastolic pressure is the level at which the pulse can no longer be heard.

the end of a hose. If you partially close the nozzle or put your finger over the end of the opening, the pressure in the hose increases. If you open the nozzle wide, the water pressure in the hose decreases and flow increases. [2] Similarly, when your arterioles narrow, it becomes more difficult for the blood to pass through them. Your heart must then work harder.

What Causes High Blood Pressure?

The causes of about 90 percent of high blood pressure cases are unknown. Such cases are called essential **hypertension**. There are risk factors that make it more or less likely for a person to develop high blood pressure. The risk factors include:

Hypertension: The medical term for abnormally high blood pressure.

Table 2.1 Blood Pressure in Adults Aged 18 Years and Older*

Blood Pressure Reading	Category	Recommended Follow-up
Diastolic Reading		
< 85	Normal blood pressure	Recheck within 2 years
85–89	High-normal blood pressure	Recheck within 1 year
90–104	Mild hypertension	Confirm within 2 months
105–114	Moderate hypertension	Evaluate or refer promptly to source of care within 2 weeks
≥ 115	Severe hypertension	Evaluate or refer immediately to source of care
Systolic Reading When Diastolic < 90		
< 140	Normal blood pressure	Recheck within 2 years
140–159	Borderline isolated systolic hypertension	Confirm within 2 months
≥ 160	Isolated systolic hypertension	Evaluate or refer promptly to source of care within 2 weeks

*Classification based on the average of two or more readings on two or more occasions.

Source:"1988 Report of the Joint National Committee on Detection, Evaluation and Treatment of High Blood Pressure," *Archives of Internal Medicine,* Vol. 148, May 1988, pp. 1023, 1038.

A chart provides guidelines on what constitutes normal and high blood pressure. Blood pressure should be checked at least once every 2 years; high levels will require more frequent tests.

- *Heredity:* Research has shown that people whose parents or close blood relatives have high blood pressure are more likely to develop hypertension.
- *Gender:* Until age 55, men are much more likely to develop high blood pressure than women. After menopause, a woman's risk of high blood pressure increases, but older men are still more likely to suffer hypertension than older women. [3]
- *Age:* As a person grows older, his or her risk of hypertension increases. Some people develop hypertension in their teens and 20s. More often, men tend to develop hypertension after age 35. Women are more likely to develop hypertension after age 45 or after menopause.
- *Race:* Studies have shown that black Americans have a greater tendency to develop high blood pressure and have more severe high blood pressure than white Americans. [4]

(continued on p. 34)

If your family has a history of high blood pressure

If your parents and other relatives have had high blood pressure, there's a good chance that you have it or may develop it, too. And if you have it, it's quite possible that your children may also develop it. Like adults, children should have regular blood-pressure checks.

The cure for high blood pressure

High Blood Pressure: Things to Consider

There isn't any. Not yet, anyway. But the important thing is that high blood pressure is controllable. To control your blood pressure, you've got to participate as part of a health-care team. Your doctor, nurse, and other team members can't do it alone—and neither can you. You must all work together.

You may have to take medication every day, perhaps for the rest of your life. And there may be other treatments, such as losing weight, using less salt, and getting more exercise.

But think about the possible consequences of untreated high blood pressure. Don't take life-or-death chances with a disease you can control.

It's no mystery

Taking blood pressure is simple and quick. The cuff placed on your arm records the two measurements in a blood-pressure reading: the pressure when your heart beats (systolic pressure) and the pressure between heartbeats (diastolic pressure).

Systolic (the first number) is the higher pressure and measures how hard your heart works to pump blood.

Diastolic (the second number) is the pressure that the arteries exert on the blood as it flows through them.

Blood pressure often rises when you are nervous or excited, but normally it goes down again *almost immediately.*

Sustained elevation is abnormal. This is why physicians usually take a series of readings before treatment.

What your blood-pressure level means

Find out what your blood-pressure numbers are. A reading of 120/80 is about normal for most people.

If you have a reading of 140/90, there are three things a physician may do: continue observation to see if *high blood pressure persists;* begin non-drug treatment, such as cutting down on your salt intake and asking you to lose weight; or initiate drug therapy if there are other risk factors *or the non-drug treatment does not work.*

Remember, high blood pressure can be controlled and continued treatment can prevent premature strokes and heart attacks.

Source: Excerpted from: *What Every Woman Should Know About High Blood Pressure,* American Heart Association.

Did You Know That . . .

By age 80, nearly 25 percent of all Americans show an elevated systolic pressure, which is attributed to the loss of blood vessel flexibility as a person ages. This condition is associated with a two-fold greater risk of stroke, as well as an increased risk of heart attack.

- *Obesity:* Defined as being more than 30 percent over the ideal body weight, obesity increases the likelihood of having high blood pressure. Even if you are a little overweight but not obese, you increase your chances of having high-normal to mild-high blood pressure.
- *Salt or sodium sensitivity:* Most Americans consume far more sodium than their bodies need. People who are particularly sensitive to salt may experience an increase in blood pressure if they overindulge. Many doctors recommend that these people follow a low-sodium diet to keep this condition under control.
- *Alcohol:* Scientists are unsure of the exact way in which alcohol causes hypertension. What they do know, however, is that large amounts of alcohol consumed regularly dramatically raise blood pressure.
- *Oral contraceptives:* These increase blood pressure in some women. If a woman smokes and takes birth control pills, her risk of developing hypertension will increase several times. The risk also increases among women who take the pill and are overweight, have hypertension during pregnancy, have a family history of high blood pressure, or have a kidney condition.
- *Sedentary life-style:* Although its effect may be indirect, a sedentary life-style often leads to obesity, a known risk factor in the development of hypertension. Regular exercise helps to control weight and relieve anxiety.
- *Stress:* It is unclear whether emotional stress causes high blood pressure. It is well known that physical stress combined with exercise causes blood pressure to rise. Anger and fright, which cause the body to release adrenaline, also raise one's blood pressure and heart rate. What is not as clear, however, is the relationship between a stressful job or living situation and hypertension.

Symptoms of Hypertension
There are no consistent identifiable symptoms of hypertension. That's why it is called the "silent disease" or the "silent killer." Some people with high blood pressure will describe themselves as feeling more tense when their blood pressure is up. Others complain of headache, dizziness, or frequent nosebleeds. Although such symptoms are commonly associated with hypertension, most of the time there are no symptoms. For this reason, hypertension is best diagnosed by taking regular blood pressure readings.

(continued on p. 36)

Many people think of high blood pressure (hypertension) as a "stress disease"—the result of overwork, no exercise, too many cocktail lunches, too much smoking, bad diet, and a thousand other things we do in our tense society. The fact is, doctors don't know what causes high blood pressure except in a few rare cases. What they do know is that nearly 58 million Americans have it and nearly half are women.

What Every Woman Should Know About High Blood Pressure

And only a small portion of all those with the disease are being adequately treated.

Why does it matter? Because high blood pressure is a killer. It leads to heart failure, stroke, kidney damage, and more.

There are no reliable symptoms of high blood pressure. But as a woman, you should know about some clues that may help you deal with this disease.

If you're taking the pill

Doctors have determined that taking contraceptive pills is associated with high blood pressure in some women. This is more likely to happen if you are overweight, have had hypertension during pregnancy, or have a predisposing condition, such as mild kidney disease or a family history of high blood pressure. So it's a good idea to ask your doctor to measure your blood pressure before prescribing the pill and then to have your blood pressure checked every six months or so. *The combination of contraceptive pills and cigarette smoking may be especially dangerous in susceptible women.*

If you're pregnant

Physicians usually keep a close watch on blood pressure during pregnancy because hypertension can develop rapidly in the last three months and is dangerous to mother and baby if not treated. This kind usually disappears after delivery but if it doesn't, it should be controlled with careful, long term treatment as recommended for all other hypertension.

As for women who already have high blood pressure, pregnancy may make the condition more severe, but again, it may not. Careful treatment allows a normal pregnancy and a normal baby.

If you're overweight

Being overweight or gaining a lot of weight as a young woman *increases the possibility of developing high blood pressure.* This is one reason why it is important to maintain normal weight throughout your life.

After menopause

As a woman grows older, her chance of having high blood pressure becomes greater than a man's. Although you may have had normal blood pressure most of your life, the chance of your getting high blood pressure increases considerably after menopause.

If you're black
Nobody knows why, but studies show that black women—even very young black women—are much more susceptible to high blood pressure than white women. Not only is the disease more common among black women, but it often tends to be more serious. In fact, one in every three black Americans over 18 is estimated to have high blood pressure.

Source: American Heart Association.

The damage done by untreated hypertension occurs in the heart and blood vessels. High blood pressure requires the heart to work harder. This in turn causes the heart muscle to increase in size or the heart's chambers to dilate, or both. Minimal enlargements may not damage a heart severely, but dramatic size increases may decrease its efficiency. Eventually, it may not be able to keep up with the body's demands.

Damage to the arteries also occurs. The arteries and arterioles become hardened (less elastic) because of the elevated blood pressure. As we discussed in the last chapter, high blood pressure

Ten Commandments for the Patient with High Blood Pressure

1. Know your blood pressure. Have it checked regularly.
2. Know what your weight should be. Keep it at that level or below.
3. Don't use excessive salt in cooking or at meals; avoid salty foods.
4. Eat a lowfat diet according to American Heart Association recommendations.
5. Don't smoke cigarettes.
6. Take your medicine exactly as prescribed; don't run out of pills even for a single day.
7. Keep your appointments with the doctor.
8. Follow your doctor's advice about exercise.
9. Live a normal life in every other way.
10. Make certain your parents, brothers, sisters, and children have their pressures checked regularly.

Source: American Heart Association.

FIGURE 2.4
Antihypertensives and Their Effects

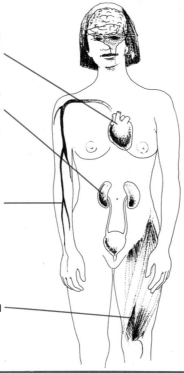

Beta-blockers reduce the force of the heartbeat and can also inhibit the dilation of the blood vessels surrounding the brain.

Diuretics increase the normal kidney action by removing excessive water from the blood. This lowers blood pressure by reducing the total volume of blood.

ACE inhibitors block enzyme activity in the blood vessels which allows the blood vessels to dilate.

Calcium channel blockers relax the muscles surrounding the blood vessels, reducing constriction.

High blood pressure can be treated with a variety of drug therapies. Antihypertensive drugs lower blood pressure either by reducing the blood volume or by dilating the blood vessels.

significantly increases the risk of atherosclerosis. Experts do not yet know why this occurs, but they do not dispute that it happens. The consequence of damage to the arteries may be heart attack, stroke, or kidney disease, depending on which arteries are most affected.

Treating Hypertension for Life: Diet, Exercise, Medications

Treating hypertension usually involves a combination of changes in life-style and administration of medication. As we noted above, some risk factors for hypertension can be modified: obesity, for

(continued on p. 41)

Treating High Blood Pressure

High blood pressure has to be treated. But once you've said that, two important questions remain: how high is high? and how do you treat it?

The toll taken by high blood pressure is well documented: heart disease and strokes leading to early death. When blood pressure is unequivocally high, treatment is clearly protective. But when it is only somewhat elevated, side effects of certain drugs may, under certain circumstances, outweigh the advantage of treatment.

There is evidence that this is the case in one specific group of people: those who, in addition to mildly elevated blood pressure, have some heart disease, as evidenced by abnormalities in the EKG. Such people may actually be harmed by the diuretics that have commonly been used, either alone or in combination with other drugs, to lower blood pressure. And it is not altogether clear that these drugs produce much benefit for otherwise healthy people who have only mild elevations of blood pressure.

Even before 1985, when these problems were highlighted by results from the Medical Research Council study in Great Britain and the Multiple Risk Factor Intervention Trial (MRFIT) in the United States, views had begun to change about the approach termed "stepped care," which had been more or less standard for over a decade. Stepped care begins with a thiazide diuretic and then, if blood pressure remains high, adds a beta-blocker. A third drug is used if blood pressure remains resistant to the first two.

Stepped care was questioned as an automatic formula for treating high blood pressure because (1) thiazide diuretics and beta-blockers have some important limitations when used as antihypertensives, and (2) attractive alternatives were coming onto the market.

Stumbling on stepped care

Perhaps the major stumbling block in treating high blood pressure has been the reluctance of people to continue therapy once they begin. Some of this is undoubtedly human cussedness. No matter how well-intentioned, most of us have difficulty maintaining daily routines that are good for us, such as flossing teeth, exercising, or taking medication according to a prescription. But another important reason has been that people simply don't feel as well after beginning medication as before.

Thiazide diuretics often produce a feeling of malaise. Some of this comes about because these drugs cause the body to lose potassium, which is vital to all kinds of normal cellular activity. Potassium supplements can (and in most cases should) be taken with the thiazides. Even with supplements, though, the body's potassium supply may become insidiously depleted, leading to episodes of weakness or to more serious problems. And the thiazides sometimes make people feel unwell quite apart from their effects on potassium.

The thiazides have other metabolic effects, which can aggravate conditions such as diabetes, gout, or kidney disease, and the fact that these drugs can raise blood cholesterol raises the question of whether they are contributing to atherosclerosis.

Even more than thiazides, beta-blockers are likely to interfere with the sense of well-being. Their range of side effects comes mainly from the fact that they interfere with the action of the sympathetic nervous system. These drugs often cause fatigue or depression. Libido may be reduced in both men and women, and men sometimes experience impotence. Susceptible people may have asthma attacks when they are put on beta-blockers, and in patients with weakened hearts these drugs can bring on heart failure.

Physicians have commonly failed to recognize how much the unpleasant effects of these standard drugs affect their patient's sense of well-being. This point was nicely documented in a British study published in 1982. Physicians, patients, and relatives of patients were asked to rate the results of antihypertensive treatment. All the doctors felt their patients were "improved." Only half the patients agreed. And only one relative in 75 said the patient had improved; the other 74 thought the patient was worse. The physicians were going solely by their measurement of blood pressure; since therapy brought their patients' blood pressures down to normal, they were more than satisfied. The patients, on the other hand, were all too conscious of the fact that they didn't feel as well as they did before they were treated. And the relatives, who had to put up with the patients' irritability, were utterly unimpressed by the "success" of this therapy.

Looking up

The quality of life while taking the older medications for blood pressure was clearly preferable to the quality of life after a stroke, but moment to moment it didn't feel that great. This situation may now be changing.

Two entirely new drug types have been introduced in the past seven years—calcium channel blockers and ACE inhibitors. There are two reasons for being pleased about this. For many people, these drugs have fewer and milder side effects than their predecessors. But also it is helpful simply to have more choices; people who tolerate one type of drug poorly may well do better with another. The opportunity to experiment with alternatives is a real advantage.

Pressure within an artery is controlled by the contraction and relaxation of tiny muscles within the artery wall. In order to contract, these vascular muscles require an inward flow of calcium from the fluid around them. The *calcium channel blockers* do just what their name implies. They attach to the surface membrane of vascular muscle at points where calcium can enter. The drug thus prevents entry of calcium and the subsequent chain reaction leading to contraction.

Calcium channel blockers act mainly on muscles in the cardiovascular system. They have relatively little effect on other parts of the body and thus have fewer side effects than the majority of antihypertensive drugs. But they do have side effects: dizziness, swelling of the ankles, headaches, palpitations, or flushing are relatively common. Most frequently prescribed for hypertension are verapamil (Calan, Isoptin) and nifedipine (Procardia). A long-action form of diltiazem (Cardizem) was approved for use in hypertension in 1988.

The calcium channel blockers have been coming into their own since the late 1970s. And since the mid-1980s yet another, completely different, type of drug has been rapidly gaining favor in treatment of high blood pressure: the so-called *ACE inhibitors.* The "ACE" in question is an enzyme found mainly in the lungs; it is responsible for activating angiotensin, a hormone, which is one of the body's major signals to increase blood pressure. Secreted by the kidneys, angiotensin arrives in the lungs, where angiotensin-converting enzyme (ACE) turns it on.

The ACE inhibitors are designer molecules developed specifically to attach to their target enzyme and prevent it from activating angiotensin. Virtually the only thing these drugs do in the body is to interact with ACE. However, ACE is not a very specific enzyme; it acts on hormones besides angiotensin. As a consequence, ACE inhibitors may lead to some side effects unrelated to blood pressure. High doses of these drugs were prescribed when they were first introduced. At these doses adverse effects were sometimes severe: impaired kidney function, diminished production of blood cells, or rashes. Current practice favors lower doses, which produce relatively few side effects. Dizziness or light-headedness, particularly when one rises to a standing position, is a predictable consequence of any medication tending to lower blood pressure. ACE inhibitors may also produce an altered sensation of taste and sometimes cause a persistent cough—both irritating but not necessarily disabling effects. Mild and often transitory rashes sometimes occur.

Most importantly, the general sense of well-being is usually not diminished by ACE inhibitors, nor do these drugs cause impotence or diminish libido. Captopril (Capoten) and enalapril (Vasotec) are the ACE inhibitors in common use; lisinopril (Zestril or Prinivil) has recently been introduced. Many physicians now prefer to use ACE inhibitors as the first drug to treat newly diagnosed high blood pressure.

Baby and bath water

The newer drugs have not done away with the older ones, if only because of cost considerations. Many people achieve good control of blood pressure without adverse effects by taking a thiazide or beta-blocker; they have no reason to change to a newer agent.

For that matter, when certain diseases coexist with high blood pressure, the older drugs may be preferable. For example, beta-blockers control angina and thus are often a good choice for a person with both angina and high blood pressure. If fluid retention accompanies hypertension, then use of a diuretic makes sense.

An important point about the thiazide diuretics is that they have their maximum effect on blood pressure at relatively low doses. Increasing the dose only increases the risk of adverse effects; it does not produce better control of pressure.

Lifestyle changes

High blood pressure does not always have to be treated with drugs. A variety of nonpharmacologic approaches can be tried, though these are most likely to work when hypertension is mild. For many people, medication will still be required, but it may be possible to use a lower dose and thus experience even fewer side effects.

Losing excess weight is probably the most important step to take. The best strategy for weight control would combine regular aerobic exercise with a low-fat diet, both of which tend to lower blood pressure in their own right. Reducing alcohol intake to two drinks a day or less is another important measure.

High salt intake seems to play a relatively minor role in *causing* high blood pressure, although the matter is still somewhat controversial. Once hypertension has become established, however, salt restriction can help with *control*. But, in and of itself, reducing salt intake, short of really drastic restriction, is rarely adequate to normalize high blood pressure. Limiting total salt intake to less than 4.5 grams a day, about half the average American's intake, will permit 50% of the people who do so to reduce their dose of medication; the other 50% will not respond. Only about half the people who try cutting their salt intake succeed, and in the ensuing weeks or months, many of them will inadvertently allow their intake to rise. So, all in all, salt restriction seems worth a try. But its effect should be monitored and expectations of success kept realistic.

Monitoring, in this case, has two parts. First, the actual salt intake should be measured. There are various, more or less cumbersome, more or less accurate ways to do this, but they all depend on measuring or estimating daily sodium excretion in the urine (which is equal to daily sodium intake). Second, blood pressure should be tracked; if it doesn't respond, then salt restriction is pointless.

One final note: Smokers should quit. This injunction is crucial with high blood pressure, because the combination of smoking and hypertension is particularly deadly.

Comfort and cost

Although it is a cliché, the phrase "silent killer" is aptly applied to hypertension. The disease does virtually all of its damage before any symptoms are experienced. And that characteristic has tended to undermine efforts at treatment, along with the fact that most of the medications available to control hypertension have made the people who took them less comfortable than they were before. The sudden onset of impotence is likely to diminish any man's enthusiasm for therapy. Such symptoms as lassitude, dizziness, nausea, and headache, however mild, lower the quality of life in the present, even though the drugs causing them promise to prolong the future. It's no surprise that noncompliance with treatment has been identified as the major limiting factor in the national effort to combat hypertension.

None of this should be taken to detract from the importance of treating high blood pressure. But the issue of compliance does complicate treatment plans. Fortunately, there's every reason to think that the quality of a hypertensive's life can be maintained in both the short and longer term, thanks to the variety of treatments now available.

The newer drugs have made a major contribution. When the rate at which patients drop out of blood pressure treatment was measured in a recent study, it was found that 13% of those on beta-blockers left treatment, but only 8% of those on ACE inhibitors. With methyldopa, an older agent, the drop-out rate was even higher, at 20%. The calcium channel blockers were not evaluated in this study, but probably are about comparable to the ACE inhibitors.

Adequate control of high blood pressure with a minimum of side effects requires close cooperation between physician and patient. Patients should never stop medication or change dosage on their own. On the other hand, they should expect close and sympathetic monitoring by the doctor, who can take advantage of the flexibility afforded by the range of available options in treatment. If one drug is poorly tolerated, nowadays there are others to try. And after a period of good control patients being treated for mild to moderate hypertension can often have their drug dose reduced.

Those who have dropped out of treatment in years past because of side effects should call their doctors to ask about the newer options. Currently, a remaining drawback of the newer drugs is relatively high cost. Treating blood pressure with a diuretic alone can cost as little as 9 cents a day; with a beta-blocker it can be as little as 42 cents. But the cost with a calcium channel blocker or ACE inhibitor is more likely to be $2.00 a day. In time, these costs are likely to come down.

Source: "High Blood Pressure: Newer Treatments," *Harvard Medical School Health Letter,* January 1989, pp. 1–4.

example; excessive salt consumption; over-indulgence in alcohol; and a sedentary life-style. All of these factors can be modified, the first three by a change in diet and the last by adopting new behavior. Fad diets are not helpful and may even be detrimental to your health. Consult your doctor before following any of them. Regardless of the diet plan you select, remember that dietary change is best undertaken in small steps over long periods of time.

Exercise may be helpful to those with hypertension. Aerobic activities, such as jogging, brisk walking, bicycling, swimming, and racket sports, increase the consumption of oxygen in the body and are thus beneficial. Exercise may also help to maintain normal body weight. Note, however, that significantly elevated blood pressure should be controlled with medication before starting a vigorous exercise program.

Many people have high blood pressure even after they have minimized all modifiable risk factors. In general, these people require medication. Many different kinds of drug therapy are used to treat high blood pressure. The exact actions and side effects differ with each class of drugs. **Diuretics** have long been used to decrease blood pressure. Today **beta-blockers** are used to decrease heart rate and blood pressure and to decrease the work load on the heart. **ACE inhibitor** medications block an enzyme that normally converts a molecule produced by the kidney into a signal to elevate blood pressure. Blocking the enzyme results in

Diuretics: Medications that allow the kidneys to excrete more salt and, consequently, more water than usual.

Beta-blockers: Drugs that simultaneously decrease the heart's rate and contraction strength and increase bronchial muscle tone.

ACE inhibitor: Medication that inhibits the action of a specific enzyme and thereby blocks one of the stages in a chain of biochemical reactions controlling blood pressure. ACE inhibitors are used to treat hypertension and heart failure.

Calcium channel blockers: Medications that block the movement of calcium across the cell membranes of arterial muscle cells, with the result that the muscles relax and blood pressure decreases.

Thrombus: A blood clot that forms within a blood vessel.

Plaque: A raised area on the inner lining of an artery wall consisting of low-density lipoproteins, cellular debris, cholesterol, and sometimes calcium; such deposits tend to form in areas of relatively turbulent blood flow, e.g., the coronary arteries.

Carotids: Arteries in the neck leading to the brain.

Embolism: A blockage of an artery caused by a clump of material (embolus) circulating in the bloodstream; embolisms are named after the affected part of body; cerebral embolisms affect the blood supply to the brain, pulmonary embolisms affect the blood supply to the lungs, and so forth.

the active molecule being present in lesser amounts. **Calcium channel blockers** are also used to control blood pressure. They work differently from beta-blockers, but both have an added advantage, that of helping to control angina. The criteria used to choose one medication over another are based on such factors as the effectiveness of a particular drug on a particular person, other associated illnesses, the drug's side effects, and the cost of the medication.

STROKE

High blood pressure can lead not only to heart trouble but also to stroke. In the United States, nearly 500,000 strokes occur each year, resulting in 150,000 deaths. In the United States, strokes are the third most common cause of death, after heart disease and cancer.

What Is a Stroke? Embolism, Thrombus, and Hemorrhage
Recall that arteries carry oxygen- and nutrient-rich blood to the tissues of the body. If the flow of blood to a specific area of the body is interrupted even for only a few minutes, the affected tissue dies. A stroke occurs when arterial blood to a portion of the brain is interrupted and the tissue fed by that artery dies, forming a scar. There are three common forms of stroke:

- **Thrombus**: Atherosclerosis, again, is the accumulation of cholesterol and cellular debris in the lining of the arteries. These substances, called **plaque**, may affect the **carotids**, major arteries in the neck that supply the brain with blood, or the arteries within the brain themselves. Atherosclerotic plaque disturbs blood flow in the artery, an ideal condition for a blood clot, or thrombus, to form. If a blood clot forms and completely blocks the artery to the brain, a stroke occurs. The victim's loss of function reflects the portion of the brain that was affected by the stroke.
- **Embolism**: A blood clot may form in the bloodstream and travel to the brain. This is called a cerebral embolism. The result is the same as with a thrombus, but the origin of the blood clot may differ. Where could a blood clot come from? If the heart is enlarged or if there is an abnormal heart rhythm, it may have formed in the heart. Or a portion of the cholesterol or atherosclerotic plaque in the arteries leading to the brain can dislodge and travel to the brain. Either can cause an embolic stroke.

FIGURE 2.5
Cerebral Embolism

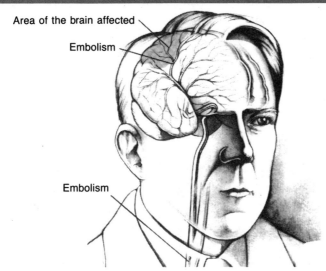

Area of the brain affected

Embolism

Embolism

Source: *1991 Heart and Stroke Facts,* American Heart Association.

A cerebral embolism is an embolism that blocks the flow of blood to some portion of the brain. Such blockages usually occur when a wandering clot (embolus) is carried by the bloodstream until it lodges in an artery leading to or in the brain.

- **Hemorrhage**: Hemorrhaging in the brain is also called a stroke because it interrupts the blood supply to brain tissue. Occasionally the wall of an artery may contain a weakness called an **aneurysm**. It is rarely a problem in childhood, but with age the weakness (if one exists) may become more pronounced. At some point the wall becomes so weak that blood begins to leak. High blood pressure puts extra strain on the artery, making a hemorrhage more likely. A leaking artery interferes with the normal flow of blood. After a while, the blood starts to occupy space in the brain intended for brain tissue. As the blood pushes the normal tissue out of the way, the tissue may die from lack of space or the leaking blood may compress the artery and cause a stroke.

Whether a stroke is caused by a thrombus, an embolus, or a hemorrhage, the effect is the same: The brain tissue that is fed by

Hemorrhage: Uncontrollable, excessive bleeding.

Aneurysm: A weakening of an artery wall.

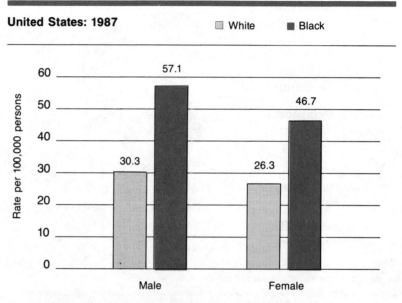

FIGURE 2.6
Age-Adjusted Stroke Death Rates

United States: 1987 □ White ■ Black

Source: American Heart Association, *1991 Heart and Stroke Facts*, p. 24.

A comparison of stroke death rates, according to race and gender. Black males have more than twice the chance of suffering a fatal stroke as do white females.

the affected artery dies. Because different sections of the brain regulate different body functions, the area of the body affected by a stroke will depend on the part of the brain in which the stroke occurs. A victim can be left with a loss of speech, weakness in one hand or in one hand and foot on the same side of the body, emotional disability (larger swings in emotions than a situation calls for, such as inappropriate laughing, crying, or depression), or loss of vision. Each brain hemisphere controls the opposite side of the body, so that if the stroke occurs on the left side of the brain, the resulting weakness will be on the body's right side.

The brain does have an amazing capacity to recover. Different areas of the brain may take over some or all of the functions of the damaged part; brain cells do not regenerate after they have died. Recuperation from a stroke may also involve learning new ways to do things, such as relearning to speak or to walk, or learning how to conduct daily activities from a wheelchair.

Predisposing Factors

The risk factors for stroke include a previous diagnosis of atherosclerotic vascular disease, smoking, hypertension, age, and being black (increased incidence in blacks most likely results from the race's relatively high incidence of hypertension). [5] An additional factor is an elevated **hematocrit**, which occurs when excessive red blood cells are found in the blood, making it thicker and more difficult to pump through small arteries. Heredity, stress, and obesity are also suspected, but they haven't been proven to be definite risk factors.

Warning Symptoms of a Stroke

Although strokes can occur without warning, some warning signs to watch for are:

1. Sudden, temporary weakness or numbness of the face, an arm, or a leg

2. Temporary difficulty with or loss of speech, or trouble understanding speech

3. Sudden, temporary dimness or a loss of vision, particularly in one eye

4. An episode of double vision

5. Unexplained headaches or a change in the pattern of headaches

6. Temporary dizziness or unsteadiness

7. A recent change in personality or mental ability. [6]

Treating a Stroke

When warning signs of a stroke occur, seek medical attention. To determine if there is arterial blockage, your physician may want to do special tests to look closely at your blood vessels. Ultrasound may be used to look for a narrowing of the carotid arteries or to look for blood clots in the heart. Administering a special dye and X-raying the arteries leading to and within the brain can pinpoint an aneurysm.

Medications that lessen the blood's ability to clot are used to prevent strokes. *Platelet cells* in the blood help blood to clot. If the platelets are inhibited, a clot is less likely to form. The most common anti-platelet drug is aspirin. Doctors can also prescribe medications that inhibit blood clot formation.

Once a stroke has occurred, treatment is directed both at

Did You Know That . . .

The American Heart Association estimated the cost of cardiovascular disease in 1990 to be $94.5 billion.

Hematocrit: Shorthand label for a measurement of the number of red blood cells in a blood sample as determined by a procedure involving a specialized centrifuge known as a hematocrit; also known as hematocrit value.

FIGURE 2.7
Areas of the Body Affected by Stroke

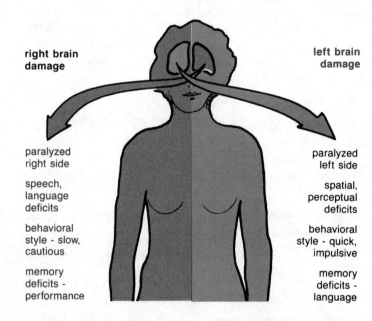

right brain
damage

left brain
damage

paralyzed
right side

speech,
language
deficits

behavioral
style - slow,
cautious

memory
deficits -
performance

paralyzed
left side

spatial,
perceptual
deficits

behavioral
style - quick,
impulsive

memory
deficits -
language

Source: American Heart Association, *1991 Heart and Stroke Facts*, p. 25.

Strokes can occur anywhere in the brain. This figure lists the effects associated with stroke damage to either the right or left side of the brain.

recovering from the stroke and preventing another stroke. The speed of recovery depends upon several factors:

• The specific area of the brain damaged
• The amount of brain tissue lost
• The rehabilitation services available to the stroke patient
• The attitude of the patient.

Rehabilitation needs to start as soon as possible after a stroke occurs if both goals are to be accomplished.

Preventing a Stroke
The best way to avoid a stroke is to actively prevent it from

(continued on p. 49)

The Long Haul

My sister-in-law, Ronnie, is a 44-year-old screen-writer and mother of two who suffered a major stroke 18 months ago. A tiny blood vessel in the brain had ruptured; she became slightly un-steady at first, and her tongue felt a bit thick. But she worsened so fast that within a week she had been hospitalized, and rapidly became paralyzed and comatose. Her son, Jeremy, then 7, had come to see her as though it might be the last time. Even more unusual than her type of stroke was the form of treatment selected for her—brain surgery. Two weeks after the operation, she could only open and close her eyes and weakly squeeze a hand. She was aware of our pres-ence—she would blink once for yes and twice for no—but just how far this awareness went, we don't know—even now. She stayed in that condi-tion for weeks.

Nobody really had much hope. One neurolo-gist, who had been dubious about the surgery in the first place, thought the not-unlikely outcome for her would be essentially worse than death—a lifetime in bed, eating and breathing through tubes. But at that time her husband fixed on a vision: Ronnie in a wheelchair at home, not doing much of anything for herself, but able to follow the growth of her children, accept their hugs and kisses after school, sit with the family at dinner. "That's all I'm hoping for," he said.

That hope has been far exceeded. Ronnie is at home, writing again, and the pages of a screen-play, commissioned by Jessica Lange before the stroke, are piling up almost miraculously. A com-puter with a large screen and a large-type printer has become the focus of much of her daily life.

"This is not make-work therapy," her husband, also a screenwriter, says. "This is real."

Not day by day, maybe not week by week, but month by month she has learned to focus her eyes, to talk again, to control her hands, to walk. Donna, an attendant who recently left nursing school to prepare for medical school, helps her out of her chair, and they make the circuit through the den, sunlit kitchen and down the hall

to the computer. This event with four-pointed cane somehow reminds me of the world's Olym-pic candidates dashing, leaping, twisting in prac-tice for what they will try in 1992. For Ronnie, the effort is every bit as intense, and will take as long. And in her way she, like them, is pushing against the frontiers of human motivation and achievement.

As such, she is part of an important new concept of rehabilitation medicine: greater and more carefully researched attention to long-term stroke therapy. Traditionally, the treatment of brain, nerve and spinal-cord damage has been divided into "acute" and "post-acute" phases—the first dealing with the immediate medical con-sequences of the damage and the need to stabi-lize the patient; the second, some weeks later, consisting of a few months of physical, occupa-tional and speech therapy.

Generally, studies on the effects of long-term stroke therapy have not been conclusive, and some neurologists remain skeptical about the need for it. After hearing, for the 100th time, the story of actress Patricia Neal's struggle back to health after her major stroke, one commented, "For all we know, Patricia Neal could have been hanging in a closet for two years and had the same recovery." In other words, long-term ther-apy can be expensive and difficult and painful; so, if we haven't proved it does any good, why bother? Well, there is now increasing evidence that long-term stroke therapy should be more aggressively pursued than it has been. Half a million people suffer strokes in the United States each year—and about 300,000 of them survive. It is becoming apparent that hundreds of thou-sands of stroke victims might improve their qual-ity of life with proper long-term therapy.

Indeed, attempts to improve on the under-standing and administration of that therapy are now being made. In the forefront of these efforts is the Neuromuscular Retraining Clinic, at the University of Wisconsin-Madison Medical School, run by Richard Balliet and Paul Bach-y-Rita, whose interest deepened after his own father, a 65-year-old college professor, suffered a stroke in the brain stem. Recovery was apparently full, but it took at least five years and a five-hour-a-day exercise program designed by his son George, then a medical student.

Several months after the stroke, Bach-y-Rita says, his father "could lift his arm over the typewriter, visually position his arm so that the middle finger was above the desired key, and then drop his arm, striking the key. Thus, using very gross movements, and with many errors, he was able to begin to type." Three years after the stroke, he returned to work. Four years after that, at the age of 72, he died of an unrelated cause, a heart attack, while mountain hiking. But perhaps the most remarkable fact, one that heightens science's interest in the case, was that the brain was examined at autopsy and extensive damage was still very much in evidence. The man was hiking in full vigor with a half-cubic-centimeter hole in a key portion of his brain known as the pons—enormous for that region—and with extensive degeneration leading out from it. How could he possibly have recovered?

As Bach-y-Rita realized, his father's case illustrates how little we understand about brain healing. Nerve cells, as far as we know, do not replace themselves once they are killed off. Extensions of the surviving cells—the "wiring" by which they send messages—can regenerate to some extent. But getting those old connections right again—crucial circuitry initially formed in the tiny machinery of the embryo—can prove impossible. Damage in adulthood can leave them dangling.

In addition, at least two other processes may help account for long-term healing. Other undamaged portions and functions of the brain, quiescent or even redundant before the stroke, may now come into their own. They may be strengthened over the long haul and accomplish feats once performed by circuits now injured. Thus left-handed stroke victims recover better from language loss than right-handed ones because they tend to have language functions distributed more widely in the brain. And finally, the rest of the body may help out. Circumventing

brain repair, it can enable the stroke sufferer to compensate for lost functions, by using different muscles, even different senses. The increase in sensitivity of vision and smell in some people with hearing loss is an example.

These and other mechanisms can be aided by practice over time. Lots of time.

Balliet says that people who are still suffering from the effects of a stroke a year after it occurred are seriously neglected by the medical community. Prejudices abound. Long-term rehabilitation is not something most physicians view as dramatic medicine. And because research remains inconclusive, insurers and other third-party payers feel justified in pulling the therapeutic floor from under the patient after a few months have elapsed. Further, because many stroke patients are elderly, and have other serious illnesses, caretakers can become too easily convinced of the futility of extended treatment. Even the pace of recovery can deceive: a plateau in improvement, needed for consolidation of gains before a further advance is often misinterpreted as the final attainable outcome. This misjudgment can confirm itself tragically, leaving the patient needlessly stranded on the plateau.

Fortunately, those prejudices are under active attack.

In the February 1989 issue of the Archives of Physical Medicine and Rehabilitation, John V. Basmajian talks of "breaking intolerable time locks for stroke survivors"; time locks that have kept us in " 'the winter of our discontent.' " New studies in England have shown that more than 45 percent of stroke survivors are functionally independent at six months. This is hardly a hopeless condition. Authorities like Bach-y-Rita and Balliet, who start an average of nine years after the initial injury, are reversing the trend and believe in the importance for stroke victims to keep plugging, working and exercising over the long term. They are not indulging in the overoptimism of those who preach "positive thinking" for treatment of advanced cancer, for example; exercise has been clearly shown to stimulate nerve function and growth, and attitude is known to make a difference for brain rehabilitation. But the rehabilitation experts now concede that it is high time for better research to show precisely what kind and how much therapy produces precisely what measure of results.

With this need in mind, Balliet, Bach-y-Rita and their colleagues are pioneering new techniques of rehabilitation—they emphasize slow movement and exacting home programs—and are carefully studying the results with up-to-date measures of muscle, nerve and brain activity. In addition to intensive physical and occupational therapies, they specialize in problems of balance and in special retraining of facial muscles. And new techniques are being employed to teach stroke victims to walk again. Few will be as lucky as Bach-y-Rita's father, but many will show significant improvement after years on a plateau.

It has now been more than a year since Ronnie was discharged from the hospital, and she has made an astounding recovery. Yet, in an important sense, it is only the beginning. No one can say just how much more recovery is in store for her; the answer lies in unsolved mysteries of the brain. But relative youth, exceptional motivation, good doctors and therapists and a supportive family are on her side—along with the new outlook in rehabilitation: long-term improvements should be *expected.*

And this is a field in which expectations can become self-fulfilling prophecies.

Balancing herself between her better leg and her cane, leaning only occasionally on Donna for support, Ronnie comes down the stretch of the long smooth wooden hallway, heading for her computer. Donna—intelligent, caring, firm, not without humor—says brightly: "Just three more steps, Ronnie. That's it. That's beautiful. Just three . . . more . . . steps."

Source: Melvin Konner, *New York Times Magazine,* 9 July 1989, pp. 55–56.

---

occurring. Preventive measures have their best results when started at an early age. Throughout adulthood, regular medical evaluation for the risk factors is also valuable protection. Beyond this standard preventive technique, some special precautions to lower one's risk factors are in order:

1. Following a low-fat, low-cholesterol, calorie-controlled diet to maintain normal body weight and normal blood cholesterol levels is very helpful in preventing premature atherosclerosis.

2. Checking blood pressure regularly, at least once every two years, is recommended. People with a personal or a familial history of borderline or high blood pressure require more frequent checkups. Those with hypertension require regular medical checkups to ensure that blood pressure is controlled.

3. Diabetics are at greater risk of developing a stroke and should be monitored to control blood sugar and blood pressure levels and for the warning signs of a stroke.

4. Routine blood tests, such as a complete blood count, can identify the problem of an elevated hematocrit. That condition, too, can be treated.

5. Oral contraceptives increase slightly the risk of stroke. Women who take oral contraceptives and are over 35 years old, especially if they also smoke, are at greater risk of stroke. These women should receive frequent screening checkups.

HEART DISEASE FROM OTHER CAUSES

Heart disease does not always result from atherosclerosis. There are other significant types of heart disease that deserve mention:

Rheumatic heart disease: Damage done to the heart, usually to the valves, by the inflammation associated with rheumatic fever.

- **Rheumatic Heart Disease**: Rheumatic fever is an inflammatory condition that affects many different tissues in the body. Frequently the heart and heart valves are involved. The cause is often a **strep infection**, commonly signaled by a sore throat or an earache, that has gone untreated. It usually affects children aged 5 to 15 and is preventable by appropriate treatment of the infection with antibiotics. The long-term effects of rheumatic fever include scarring of the heart valves. Once scarred, they may leak or the valve opening may narrow, diminishing blood flow through the valve.

Strep infection: An infection caused by the streptococcus organism.

Congenital heart disease: Structural abnormalities of the heart that occur during development within the fetus.

- **Congenital Heart Disease**: This condition, a structural abnormality of the heart caused by defective formation of the heart chambers, valves, or vessels, occurs while the fetus is in the uterus. The cause of abnormal heart formation is not usually identifiable. It is sometimes the result of a viral infection in the mother during the first 3 months of pregnancy. **Rubella**, or the German measles, is especially dangerous and can be prevented by appropriate immunization prior to pregnancy. When congenital heart disease is diagnosed, surgery may be recommended.

Rubella: A viral infection, also known as German measles, whose usual symptoms are a mild fever and skin rash that lasts for several days, then disappears; rubella may occur at any age but most often affects children between the ages of 6 and 12; ordinarily a mild disease, rubella can have serious consequences for the fetus if contracted by a nonimmune pregnant woman.

- **Heart Failure**: **Congestive heart failure** may occur for any of several reasons. The heart muscle may be weakened by long-standing untreated hypertension. A significant portion may be damaged by a major heart attack or several heart attacks. Heart failure may also result from the heart working harder to push the blood across a narrowed valve. A chamber may enlarge if there is too much backflow from a leaking valve. Whatever the cause, the result is the same. The heart muscle weakens and the heart becomes less able to handle a normal blood volume. Fluid begins to back up in the tissues of the body. While fluid may accumulate in any tissue, the lungs are usually affected first. Excess fluid buildup in the body is especially apt to affect the legs.

Heart failure: Ineffective pumping of one side of the heart leading to a buildup of fluid within the tissues of the body, commonly in the lungs and the feet.

Congestive heart failure: Ineffective pumping of both sides of the heart, leading to a buildup of fluid within the tissues of the body.

Bacterial endocarditis: Infection in the lining of the heart and the heart valves.

- **Bacterial Endocarditis**: Systemic infections can result in bac-

(continued on p. 54)

29 Little Ways to Lower Your Blood Pressure

When it comes to high blood pressure, every point counts. Studies show that if you're hypertensive, every little incremental rise in blood pressure corresponds to a jump in your risk of heart disease and stroke. So anything you can do to nudge your blood pressure down—if only a few points—is all to the good.

To that end we present a smorgasbord of 29 techniques you can use right now to counterpunch hypertension. Experts point out that such "lifestyle strategies" have in many cases helped people to either cut back on their antihypertensive medication or drop their blood pressure into the safety zone.

Is every one of these strategies guaranteed to lower your blood pressure significantly? Not at all. Everybody is different: What works for someone else may not work for you. And though science has declared some of the techniques highly effective in reducing chronic high blood pressure, others aren't as highly rated. Some of these may push blood pressure down, but only temporarily. Or they may simply be the latest untested-yet-safe proposal for making a dent in your hypertension. The point is that if you're really serious about lowering high blood pressure, they're all worth a try, especially since every little bit of pressure-lowering helps.

So the idea is to try as many of these strategies as possible (under your doctor's supervision and as adjuncts to any medical treatment you may be undergoing). There's every reason to believe that a lot of the techniques will have a cumulative effect. They're more likely to be effective, however, if you have mild hypertension—a systolic reading (the first number) of 140–159 or a diastolic reading (the second number) of 90–104. But even higher pressures may respond to some of these strategies. Typically, though, medication is the first and most prudent therapy for people with severe hypertension—systolic of 160 or higher, or diastolic of 115 or higher.

1. Lose weight. If you're overweight, this is one of the most potent antihypertension lifestyle changes you can make. It has a proven impact: On the average, people can lose one point off both their systolic and diastolic blood pressures for every two pounds they drop.

2. Eat fish. Preliminary studies have suggested an association between eating fish or fish oil and lower blood pressure. Researchers theorize that it's the omega-3 fatty acids in ocean fish (such as mackerel, tuna and salmon) that could somehow be counteracting hypertension. The experts' recommendation: Dine on fish at least two or three times a week.

3. Go for a walk. Research shows that regular aerobic exercise (walking, cycling, swimming and the like) may lower blood pressure four or five points. How much exercise does it take? Most of the studies reporting decreases in blood pressure in hypertensives had people working out 30 to 60 minutes three times a week. (You have to work up to this level slowly, though, and with your doctor's blessing.)

4. Say when. Over the long haul, consuming more than two mixed drinks (one ounce of alcohol each), two beers or two glasses of wine a day can raise your blood pressure. The danger of lower amounts is unclear, but experts are unanimous in their recommendation: Limit the booze. Alcohol abuse has been called "the most common cause of reversible hypertension."

5. Watch the fat. The evidence is far from conclusive, but some research suggests that intake of saturated fats (prevalent in red meat, many dairy products and other foods) may be linked to rises in blood pressure. And polyunsaturated fats (prevalent in certain vegetable products like safflower and corn oil) seem to lower it. A growing mass of evidence suggests that monounsaturated fats, predominant in olive oil and a few other foods, may provide the same benefits. So experts are advocating a prudent course. First, lower your total fat intake to less than 30 percent of calories. Then keep the saturated fats to a minimum (no more than one-third of total fat), and favor the monos and polys.

7. Find your true blood pressure. Some people with high blood pressure are believed to have "white-coat hypertension." Their blood pressure rockets only when it's taken in their doctor's office. So before you make a commitment to blood-pressure medication, have your pressure measured over a full day with a portable unit. (Your doctor may loan one out.) Or have your blood pressure measured several times in a variety of settings.

7. Don't salt the water. Water softeners replace calcium and magnesium with sodium. So use your softener, just don't hook it up to the tap water used for cooking and drinking.

8. Eat a baked potato. A baked potato with no added sodium has a powerful "K Factor," says potassium expert George Webb, Ph.D., associate professor of physiology and biophysics at the University of Vermont Medical College. It has 130 times more potassium (chemical symbol: K) than sodium. Lack of potassium has been associated with an increase in blood pressure. And some researchers feel that the key thing is to maintain a 2:1 or 3:1 ratio of potassium to sodium in your diet. In general, fresh fruits and vegetables have far more potassium than sodium. Top choices: beans, rice, fresh fruits and grains. (But check with your doctor. Some people with certain kidney diseases can't tolerate extra potassium.)

9. Beware the pill. Oral contraceptives raise blood pressure slightly in most women and are estimated to cause high blood pressure in about 5 percent. So if you want to use oral contraceptives, ask your doctor about using a preparation with low estrogen-progestogen content. Low-dose formulas are less likely to have a pressure-raising effect.

10. Steam it. Boiling vegetables leaches away a good part of their potassium and magnesium (another mineral that may be linked to reduced blood pressure) and allows sodium to be picked up more easily by the food. It's even worse, of course, if you add salt. So as part of your own antihypertension campaign, microwave, steam or bake your food. Stir-frying is O.K., but use oil sparingly.

11. Pet your dog. Or your rabbit. Or your cat. Any animal that's soft and cuddly. Some researchers suspect that interacting with a pet may lower blood pressure, at least temporarily. "The minute you start talking to and petting your dog, your blood pressure goes down and stays down during the interaction," says Aline Halstead Kidd, Ph.D., professor in psychology at Mills College in Oakland, California. "The point is, human-to-human interactions make certain demands. A pet allows you to interact with another living being that makes no demands and loves you without regards to anything." It's important that the animal be yours, Dr. Kidd says. Meeting a strange pet can entail the same cautious social minuet as when you meet another person. In a 1986 survey, some 20 percent of the doctors polled thought hypertensive patients could benefit by going to the dogs.

12. Look at fish. "Anything that holds your attention so you're looking and listening but not thinking and worrying reduces blood pressure transiently," says Aaron Katcher, M.D., a psychiatrist at the University of Pennsylvania. "And this could be from watching a fireplace, taking a walk in the park, going bird-watching or watching fish in an aquarium." Based on studies of other relaxation techniques, Dr. Katcher believes that doing any of these things for 15 minutes twice a day may be an effective treatment for some people with mild hypertension.

13. Do your own stress test. Though it's possible to be perfectly calm and still have hypertension, or have normal blood pressure and be a nervous wreck, some people do react to stress with at least a temporary rise in blood pressure. And scientists suspect that stress plays a still-unknown role in chronic hypertension. So to find out for sure if stress is boosting your blood pressure, test yourself. Buy a home blood-pressure monitor and have it calibrated by your physician or pharmacist (otherwise it may be off by as much as 30 points). Your doctor can show you the proper sitting position and technique for taking your pressure. Then take your blood pressure before, during and after a stressful activity. This way you'll know if the stressful event is affecting your blood pressure and whether you should avoid it. Good news: Not all stressful or exciting situations have an effect.

14. Live with less sodium. Not everyone with high blood pressure is affected by dietary sodium (the main ingredient in salt), but most are. And you may be one of them. Excess sodium will cause sodium-sensitive people to retain more fluid, which can raise blood pressure. Hormonal changes may also contribute by constricting blood vessels. Unfortunately, there's no easy way to determine who's sodium sensitive. But most of us consume far too much sodium and could stand to cut back. So experts say reduce your total daily sodium intake to 1,500 to 2,000 milligrams—the amount you'd find in one teaspoon of salt. Even modest reductions may be enough to enable some people to reduce or even eliminate their hypertension medication.

15. Check your water. Your largest source of sodium, if you're on a sodium-restricted diet, could be a surprising one—your drinking water. It doesn't necessarily taste salty. In a 1981 study, 42 percent of the nation's water supply exceeded the Environmental Protection Agency's recommendation of 20 mg. of sodium per liter. Check your water sodium level with your local water supplier or the EPA.

16. Measure often. The regular measuring of blood pressure over time seems to help some people nudge their pressure down. One possible reason: If you're aware of your blood pressure, you may take steps (perhaps even subconsciously) that may help. Such as not dousing your baked potato with salt. Or reacting more serenely to stress.

17. Enjoy a good laugh. A hearty laugh causes a small and fleeting decrease in blood pressure. Even more important, laughter is a great way to relieve stress and anger. Go to a funny movie. Be with people who make you laugh, rather than who debate. The long-term effects of laughter on blood pressure are unknown, but certainly there are no negative side effects to laughing.

18. Use diet pills with caution. Many diet pills, both prescription and over-the-counter, contain a substance that's a mouthful—phenylpropanolamine (PPA). PPA is believed to depress the part of the brain that controls appetite. But in some people it can also raise blood pressure, among other possible side effects.

19. Select fast foods wisely. Many fast foods are loaded with sodium and fat. A McDonald's Big Mac has 950 mg. of sodium. A Burger King Whopper with cheese has 1,164 mg. of sodium, which can by itself exceed the recommended amounts for those on sodium-restricted diets.

20. Keep an anger diary. Both habitually holding anger in or lashing out without trying to solve a problem can lead to transient—and possibly chronic—increases in blood pressure. Keeping track of your anger in a diary, however, helps you identify and understand the causes of your anger. Your diary should monitor what made you angry, what you did about it, how you felt at the time and later. Then you can reflect and develop strategies for defusing anger constructively.

21. Relax from head to toe. Progressive muscle relaxation is a proven technique for relieving stress. Sit or lie in a comfortable position and tense and relax the muscles of your body in sequence. Start by clenching your fists for three or four seconds, concentrating on how the tension feels, then relax your hand muscles, letting go of the tension.

Try this tensing/relaxing sequence for all major muscles—those in your neck, shoulders, back, arms, abdomen, buttocks, thighs, calves and feet. Ideally, you'll learn to relax these muscles without tensing them first. Try this exercise for 10 minutes, twice a day.

22. Smell a slice of apple pie. Preliminary research suggests that certain scents—particularly spiced apple—may nearly double any blood-pressure benefits of quiet relaxation. One theory is that apple pie can bring back pleasant associations with holidays. The research is too inconclusive to say that a given odor will nudge your own blood pressure down. But if you want to test the notion, try a fragrance you find particularly appealing.

23. Watch for 'hidden' salt. Cured meats, such as bacon, hot dogs and sausage, are high in sodium and fat. Many (but not all) canned soups are high in sodium. So are some brands of canned tuna, prepared pancakes, some TV dinners and regular soy sauce. So become a label reader when you grocery shop.

24. Listen to music. There's no hard scientific data yet, but some music-therapy experts think that tuning in to tunes may help lower blood pressure. But what kind of music? Heavy metal? Ugh. The experts suggest that the best tunes are of the soothing kind—quiet, nonvocal, slow, with predictable rhythms.

25. Check your medication. Propranolol, a common hypertensive that slows heart rate, may limit the cardiovascular benefits of a workout, according to a study for the University of Vermont School of Medicine. One of these benefits is decreased blood pressure. (The benefits of the drug itself, of course, remain intact.) So if you exercise and are taking propranolol, ask your doctor about switching to another blood-pressure drug.

26. Talk to yourself. You can learn to respond more calmly to a stressful or anger-provoking situation by talking your way through it beforehand. For example, let's say you have to meet with someone who you know often irritates you. Instead of saying to yourself, "I'm going to lose it when he acts like a jerk," say "There's no reason to automatically assume that he'll get on my nerves. I'm going to stay relaxed. I won't get angry."

27. Work as a team. Blood pressure experts say that you're more likely to stick with any antihypertensive regimen if you enlist the whole family in the effort. Some suggestions: Do exercises that other family members can enjoy with you, like walking and bicycling. Don't keep food in the house that one person can eat but another cannot.

28. Douse that cigarette. Studies show that smokers seem to get less benefit from the pressure-lowering drug propranolol. Also, though smoking itself doesn't seem to raise blood pressure over the long run, it can damage the cardiovascular system and make the consequences of having high blood pressure worse.

29. Watch what you chew. Chew this over: Smokeless tobacco often contains large amounts of sodium for flavor and also to help the body absorb nicotine.

—*Joe Mullich*

Source: *Prevention*, June 1989, pp. 33–40.

teria entering the bloodstream. Dental work and other medical procedures may also allow bacteria into the bloodstream. When that happens, an infection of the heart valves and lining of the chambers of the heart may occur. An abnormal heart valve is more vulnerable to infection, making people with heart murmurs especially susceptible. They should seek the advice of their health-care professionals regarding the use of antibiotics to prevent infection from medical or dental procedures. People who have had rheumatic fever or have congenital heart disease are also particularly at risk for endocarditis. Users of illegal intravenous drugs are also at increased risk.

Stroke is the third most common cause of death in the United States. Nearly 1 out of every 4 Americans suffers one of its major contributing factors, hypertension. Although high blood pressure has no symptoms, it is easy to diagnose and can be treated. Controlling hypertension helps to avoid or delay serious problems associated with it, such as stroke and heart disease. Ⓦ

Cancer

CONSIDER, IF YOU WILL, some grim statistics: Cancer is the second most common cause of death in the United States. One out of 3 people develop cancer at some point in their lives, and an estimated 514,000 Americans died of cancer in 1991. Approximately 20 percent of all deaths are from cancer.

The diagnosis of cancer has always carried frightening connotations: terminal prognosis, excruciating chemotherapy, and painful demise. Recent scientific breakthroughs, however, have served to increase life expectancy for cancer patients. With early detection and proper treatment, many sufferers of cancer recover completely and lead healthy, normal lives. In addition, scientists have discovered several steps people can take to reduce their risk of contracting certain types of cancer. The causes, detection, treatment, and possible prevention of the disease are the focus of this chapter.

THE NATURE AND CAUSES OF CANCER

There is no one cause of cancer. Recently, scientists have discovered a number of mechanisms influencing cancer development in humans. One such mechanism is the lack of **contact inhibition**; another is **growth factor** production.

Normal human cells reproduce themselves to replace cells that are dying or injured. The new cell stops growing when it touches a surrounding cell. Called contact inhibition, this feedback process helps control normal growth. **Malignant or cancerous cells** (these words are used interchangeably) lack this inhibition and grow without being controlled. Research also

Contact inhibition: A natural feedback mechanism whereby a normal cell stops growing when it touches a surrounding cell.

Growth factor: Abnormal proteins that ignore natural feedback and stimulate cells to continue to grow and multiply, resulting in a tumor.

Malignant or cancerous cells: A tumor that is not confined and has a tendency to infiltrate normal tissue and metastasize.

There are approximately 30,000 new cases of oral cancer diagnosed each year. The major risk factor for oral cancer is tobacco use.

FIGURE 3.1

Total Deaths from Cancer per 100,000 Persons in the United States from 1900–1985

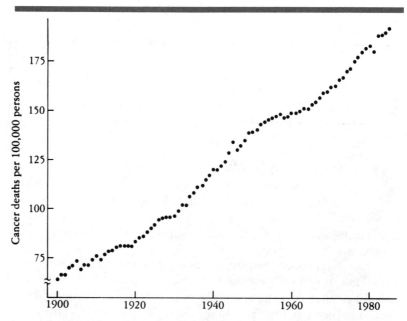

Source: D. Prescott, A. Flexer, *Cancer: The Misguided Cell* (Sunderland, MA: Sinaver Associates, 1986), p. 3.

The significant increase in deaths from cancer from the beginning of this century can partially be explained by the decrease in deaths from other causes, particularly infectious diseases.

indicates that some cells produce abnormal proteins, called growth factors, that ignore the feedback loop and stimulate the cells to continue to grow and multiply. Either results in a tumor.

A tumor is merely an abnormal growth. A **benign** tumor is one that does not spread to other tissues. It remains confined and rarely kills but could prove fatal if it interferes with normal functioning and cannot be surgically removed—as in the case of a brain tumor. A *malignant tumor*, on the other hand, has 4 characteristics that make it potentially lethal:

1. Cells originating from one abnormal stem cell, which produces a group, or clone, of malignant cells. A detectable tumor can contain 1 billion or more such cells

Benign: The opposite of malignant; a tumor that is usually encapsulated, does not infiltrate normal tissue, and does not metastasize.

2. Unregulated growth

3. Cells that do not mature and differentiate (to become a specific kind of cell and have a well-defined function—for example, a liver cell) in a normal fashion

4. Malignant cells that have the capacity to disseminate to other parts of the body, a process called **metastasis**

Most cancers occur in stages. In the initial stage, the cancer is usually confined to the site where it originated. It does, however, invade the normal tissue locally. In the next stage, it travels to nearby **lymph nodes**. In the last stage, the cancer cells metastasize to other tissues. The symptoms of individual cancers depend upon the size, location, and nature of the molecules produced by the various cancers.

THE WARNING SIGNS OF CANCER

The American Cancer Society has provided a list of 7 warning signs of cancer that should prompt a visit to your doctor. These warning signs are:

1. Change in bowel or bladder habits

2. A sore that does not heal

3. Unusual bleeding or discharge

4. Thickening or lump in the breast or elsewhere

5. Indigestion or difficulty swallowing

6. Obvious change in wart or mole

7. Nagging cough or hoarseness. [1]

If you have one or more of these warning signs, see your doctor.

TREATING CANCER

The treatment of cancer depends in part on the stage at which it is detected. Surgery may be adequate if a cancer is still localized. **Radiation treatments** (X rays) are helpful against certain cancers. **Chemotherapy**, medication directed at killing rapidly di-

Lymph nodes: Glands that produce and filter lymph, a clear fluid containing antibodies and white blood cells that circulates through the lymphatic system.

Metastasis: The movement of malignant cells to, and proliferation at, body sites other than those at which the tissue of origin was located.

Radiation treatments: The use of X rays to treat cancer.

Chemotherapy: Treatment involving the use of drugs or other medication designed to kill or reduce the growth rate of cancer cells.

viding cells, is also used to treat the disease. The natural history of a particular cancer and its sensitivity to different treatments ultimately determine the approach to be used.

THE MOST COMMON CANCERS

The incidence of cancer and the sites most commonly affected are different in women than in men. For women, 70 percent of all cancers take one of the following forms: In descending order of occurrence, these are lung cancer, breast cancer, cancer of the colon and rectum, cancer of the uterus, and leukemias and lymphomas. In men, 72 percent of all cancers occur in 5 locations: lungs, colon and rectum, prostate, urinary tract, and blood and lymph tissues. [2] Here, we will discuss first the cancers that are most preventable, followed by the cancers that are most common.

Lung Cancer

Lung cancer kills more men and women than any other form of the disease. Most people with lung cancer die within one year of diagnosis. [3] Lung cancer most often occurs in people between the ages of 55 and 65. It can, however, occur earlier in life. The greatest risk factor contributing to the development of lung cancer is cigarette smoking. People who do not smoke can also contract lung cancer, but their risk of doing so is much smaller than that of those who do smoke. Specifically, if a man smokes 2 packs of cigarettes a day for 20 years, his risk of getting lung cancer is 60 to 70 times greater than for a nonsmoking man the same age. [4] Certain occupations also increase the risk of lung cancer. Asbestos workers, for example, have an increased incidence of lung cancer. If they also smoke, their risk of developing lung cancer may be 100 times that of nonsmokers who do not work with asbestos.

The symptoms of lung cancer include a chronic cough, shortness of breath, chest pain, and blood-tinged **phlegm**. These symptoms reflect the tumor's location. Recurrent episodes of pneumonia that won't respond to treatment may also signal lung cancer. More advanced symptoms often include loss of appetite, loss of weight, nausea and vomiting, hoarseness, bone pain, and neurological problems. Lung cancer most frequently spreads to the lymph glands, bone and bone marrow, and brain. [5]

Lung cancer is often diagnosed by a combination of physical examination, chest X ray and, finally, a **biopsy**. A biopsy is essential to the diagnosis. Several different kinds of cells can cause lung cancer. Treatment and prognosis, or even an estimate

Phlegm: Mucus, especially in excessive amounts, produced by the cells lining the bronchial tree and excreted by the respiratory system.

Biopsy: Removal and microscopic examination of tissue from a living body, most frequently from a tumor, for the purpose of determining whether or not it is malignant.

FIGURE 3.2
Cancer Incidence and Deaths by Site and Sex

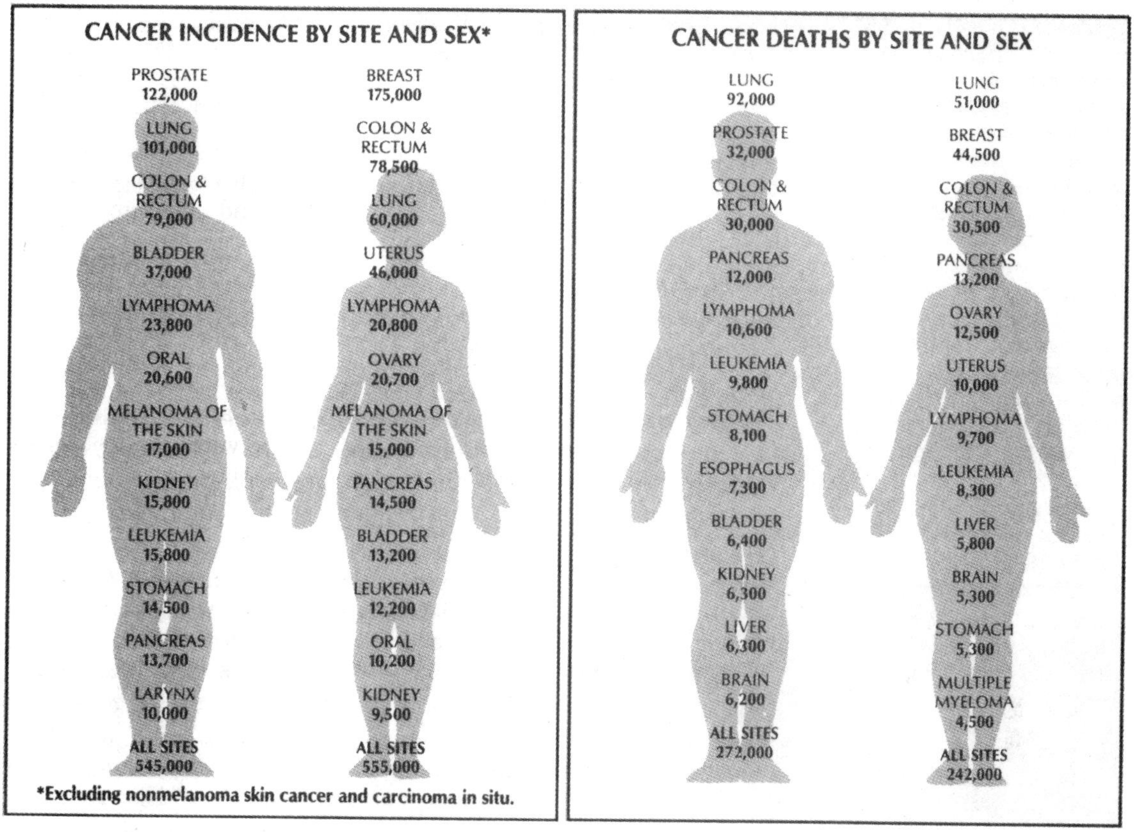

CANCER INCIDENCE BY SITE AND SEX*		CANCER DEATHS BY SITE AND SEX	
PROSTATE 122,000	BREAST 175,000	LUNG 92,000	LUNG 51,000
LUNG 101,000	COLON & RECTUM 78,500	PROSTATE 32,000	BREAST 44,500
COLON & RECTUM 79,000	LUNG 60,000	COLON & RECTUM 30,000	COLON & RECTUM 30,500
BLADDER 37,000	UTERUS 46,000	PANCREAS 12,000	PANCREAS 13,200
LYMPHOMA 23,800	LYMPHOMA 20,800	LYMPHOMA 10,600	OVARY 12,500
ORAL 20,600	OVARY 20,700	LEUKEMIA 9,800	UTERUS 10,000
MELANOMA OF THE SKIN 17,000	MELANOMA OF THE SKIN 15,000	STOMACH 8,100	LYMPHOMA 9,700
KIDNEY 15,800	PANCREAS 14,500	ESOPHAGUS 7,300	LEUKEMIA 8,300
LEUKEMIA 15,800	BLADDER 13,200	BLADDER 6,400	LIVER 5,800
STOMACH 14,500	LEUKEMIA 12,200	KIDNEY 6,300	BRAIN 5,300
PANCREAS 13,700	ORAL 10,200	LIVER 6,300	STOMACH 5,300
LARYNX 10,000	KIDNEY 9,500	BRAIN 6,200	MULTIPLE MYELOMA 4,500
ALL SITES 545,000	ALL SITES 555,000	ALL SITES 272,000	ALL SITES 242,000

*Excluding nonmelanoma skin cancer and carcinoma in situ.

Source: American Cancer Society, *Cancer Facts and Figures 1991*, p. 11.

Shown here are the most common cancers and the number of cancer deaths for both men and women, listed in descending order of occurrence.

of the probable course of the disease and outcome for the patient, depend upon knowing the cancer's cell type and extent. That is, has it metastasized, and, if so, where has it spread? In most cases of lung cancer, the interval between diagnosis and death ranges from a few months to perhaps 1 or 2 years. The 5-year survival rate after "curative surgery" is between 27 and 37 percent. [6]

Is it reasonable to have periodic chest X rays to detect lung cancer early? Thus far, studies have shown that early detection of lung cancer through X-ray screening does not increase one's chances of survival. As a result, routine chest X rays solely to look for lung cancer are not recommended. Periodic microscopic evaluation of sputum (phlegm) for cancerous cells has also been tried as a screening method. It too does not seem to change the long-term survival rate for victims of lung cancer.

Cancer and Smoking   If lung cancer is among the most lethal cancers, it is also one of the most preventable. The risk of developing lung cancer is directly related to the amount of cigarette smoke to which one is exposed. Thirty percent of all cancer deaths and about 85 percent of all lung cancer deaths can be attributed to cigarette smoking. [7]. Because of the relative increase in smoking among women, lung cancer has now surpassed breast cancer as the leading cause of cancer deaths among women.

Passive Smoking   There is increasing evidence that passive or involuntary smoking—inhaling the smoke of other people's cigarettes—is a risk factor for nonsmokers. According to the U.S. surgeon general in his 1986 report, "Cigarette smoking is an addictive behavior and the individual smoker must decide whether or not to continue that behavior; however, it is evident from the data presented that the choice to smoke cannot interfere with the nonsmoker's right to breathe air free of tobacco smoke." [8]

Since publication of this report, state and local lawmakers have enacted new policies limiting smoking in public restaurants, airlines, and offices. The new rules are designed to protect nonsmokers from the adverse effects of involuntary smoking.

Other Cancer Risks for Smokers   Cigarette smoking also increases the risk of cancer of the **larynx**, oral cavity, and **esophagus**. And, although the mechanism isn't yet known, alcohol consumed with the cigarettes amplifies the risk of cancer. Other forms of cancer associated with cigarette use include cancers of the bladder, kidney, pancreas, stomach, and uterine cervix.

Pipe and cigar smokers are less likely to inhale smoke and have fewer cases of lung cancer. However, cigarette and cigar smokers have the same mortality rates from cancers of the mouth, larynx, and esophagus—locations where both types of smoke come into contact with tissue. Smokeless tobaccos, snuff or chewing tobacco, also increase the risk of developing cancers of the mouth and throat.

Larynx: Voice box; the area surrounding and including the vocal cords.

Esophagus: The tubular structure located immediately behind the windpipe (trachea) that connects the mouth and the stomach.

FIGURE 3.3

One Cancer You Can Give Yourself

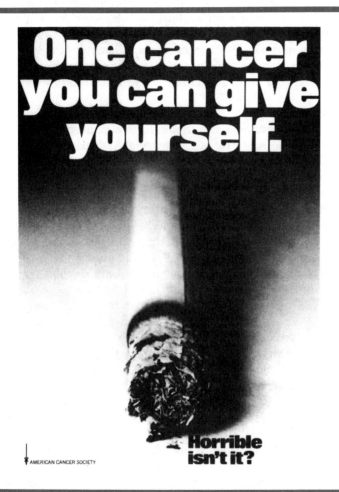

Thirty percent of all cancer deaths and almost 85 percent of all lung cancer deaths can be attributed to cigarette smoking.

Happily, if you stop smoking, your risk of developing cancer decreases. Ten years after the cessation of smoking, the risk of developing lung cancer drops to nearly the same rate as for those who have never smoked.

Current trends in smoking rates are encouraging. Only 30 percent of all people over the age of 18 now smoke cigarettes regularly, the lowest level in 40 years. Men have cut their smoking rates from nearly 42 percent in 1976 to 31 percent today. Women have reduced their smoking rates from 32 percent to 27 percent over the same period. The percentage of high school seniors who smoke cigarettes daily has decreased from 29 percent in 1976 to 18 percent in 1988. [9] Still, 29 percent of the adult population in the United States smoke. Clearly, with nearly 1 in 3 Americans still smoking cigarettes, further efforts are in order to reduce that and other forms of tobacco consumption.

Breast Cancer

Breast cancer is the most common form of cancer in women. It is the second leading cause of cancer-related deaths in women. [10] About 1 in 10 women will develop breast cancer. Although it is most common after the age of 50, some women may be stricken while still in their 20s. For reasons that are still unknown, the incidence of breast cancer has continued to climb since 1973. [11]

Breast cancer usually presents itself as a lump, a hardening or dimpling of breast tissue. It is usually, but not always, painless. Eighty to 90 percent of all breast lumps are benign. Although that is reassuring if you find a lump in your breast, you can't know if any lump is benign until further tests have been done. Final diagnosis of breast cancer has to be made with a biopsy.

Treatment of breast cancer depends on several factors. The first thing doctors usually do is remove the lump and surrounding lymph nodes, called a **lumpectomy**, or, in more advanced cases, remove the breast and surrounding lymph nodes, called a **mastectomy**. Statistics for recurrence and cure are nearly the same for both procedures. The decision as to which surgery to perform is primarily determined by the stage of the disease, which in turn often depends upon how early it has been detected. A patient's age, pre- or post-menopausal status, the extent of the cancer, and its degree of sensitivity to hormones also play a role in the type of surgery and the extent of any additional treatment. Chemotherapy immediately after surgery has been shown to increase survival rates in most breast cancer patients. X-ray treatments of the breast from which the lump was taken also increase the chance of cure and long-term survival. [12]

Chemotherapy is medication taken orally or intravenously for the treatment of cancer. It is used at two different stages of breast cancer. The initial use often occurs at the time of diagnosis. Additional use occurs if and when the disease recurs. Chemotherapy is a broad term referring to a variety of medications that

Lumpectomy: The removal of a lump, usually referring to the removal of a cancerous lump in a woman's breast without removing the breast.

Mastectomy: Surgical removal of the breast tissue.

Cigarettes Trigger Lung Cancer Gene, Researchers Find

Chemicals in cigarette smoke will switch on a gene in lung cells that then helps make those compounds far more likely to cause cancer, researchers have reported.

The gene seems to be more likely to flick on in some people than in others, the scientists said, which may partly explain why only about 7 percent of heavy smokers develop lung cancer.

The chemicals that trigger the gene are considered the most important cancer-causing compounds in cigarette smoke and in certain environmental and industrial pollutants. As a result, the researchers said, the gene may soon be useful as a marker to identify those people who are at high risk for coming down with lung cancer.

"If we could identify those people in whom this gene is easily activated, then we could counsel them, not only not to smoke, but to avoid exposure to certain environmental pollutants," said Dr. Theodore L. McLemore, the main author of the report, in [a recent] issue of the Journal of the National Cancer Institute. Dr. McLemore, formerly a researcher at the cancer institute, now heads the pulmonary medicine division for St. Joseph's Hospital in Paris, Tex.

Quitting Usually Shuts Down Gene

He said that in normal lung tissue the gene shuts down rapidly once a person gives up smoking, becoming nearly undetectable in lung cells only two weeks later. But he and his colleagues also found that in half the lung tumors they examined the gene seemed to be stuck in a permanently active position.

"Our work supports the idea that the sooner you quit smoking, the less the chance that you'll go on to develop pulmonary cancer," Dr. McLemore said.

The gene, known as CYP1A1, normally helps liver cells tear down toxins into a harmless form that the body can easily dispose of.

But the researchers said that among those in whom the gene switches on easily, it bursts to life in the lungs when pulmonary tissue is exposed to aromatic hydrocarbons, compounds found in cigarette tar and other pollutants. The gene produces an enzyme that transforms hydrocarbons into highly reactive carcinogens that damage DNA and set the stage for cancer.

The scientists said that without the transformation resulting from the enzyme, the hydrocarbons would remain as pro-carcinogens, which cannot on their own mutate DNA.

"Unless you metabolize these pro-carcinogens of smoke into their active state, you can't have the mechanism for the production of cancer," said Dr. McLemore. "So this gene must play a very important role in the cancer cascade."

But researchers warn that even [for]those people who are shown not to have an easily triggered CYP1A1 gene, smoking is by no means risk-free. "There are about ten thousand chemicals in cigarette smoke, and this gene is involved in only one class of them," said Dr. Richard E. Kouri, director of research at BIOS Corporation in New Haven and a contributor to the research. He proposes that a number of other genes are likely to be involved in the genesis and progression of lung cancer as well.

Source: Natalie Angier, *New York Times* (21 August 1990), sec. 3, p. 3.

interfere with the normal biological function of cells and destroy cells. Researchers believe that because cancerous cells grow more quickly than normal ones, they are more biologically active and therefore more vulnerable to the effects of chemotherapy. Normal cells that divide and grow quickly are most subject to the side effects chemotherapy causes. Among those affected may be blood cells—especially the ones that fight infection—which can decrease in number, and blood clotting cells (platelets). The cells lining the gastrointestinal tract are also vulnerable; loss of appetite, nausea, and vomiting are frequent side effects of chemotherapy. Hair loss also occurs. The side effects are unpleasant but are often worthwhile, for the treatment can be quite effective. For example, studies show that chemotherapy used in the initial phases of breast cancer increases the average length of survival for patients by 2 to 3 years. [13]

Radiation treatments involve beaming an external X ray onto the affected area for a few minutes at a time, 5 days a week, for about 6 weeks. Side effects include hardening, scarring, and shrinkage of the surrounding tissue. This form of therapy is used for women who choose to have a lumpectomy, as well as for those whose cancer recurs locally on the chest wall. The survival rates for women who choose lumpectomy and radiation, as well as chemotherapy when indicated, are the same as those for women who choose mastectomy.

What Are the Risk Factors for Breast Cancer? The cause of breast cancer is unknown, but doctors believe that its incidence increases with age, particularly after the age of 50. [14] Also at increased risk are those with a family history of breast cancer, women who have never had children, women whose first child was born after their 30th birthday, women with other forms of breast disease, and women who have already had breast cancer. Because breast cancer is so common, none of these risk factors need be present for a woman to develop breast cancer. Even if you have none of them, therefore, you should still be examined for breast cancer periodically.

Early Detection
Because the cause of breast cancer is unknown, its occurrence is difficult to prevent. The best protection offered, then, is early detection. Early detection improves the rate of cure and long-term survival. The 5-year survival rate for women diagnosed with localized breast cancer has increased to nearly 90 percent. If the cancer has spread, the statistics aren't nearly as favorable. Testing for breast cancer involves 3 distinct steps:

1. Breast self-examinations (BSE) monthly

2. Mammography, X-ray images of the breast. The American Cancer Society recommends that women between the ages of

(continued on p. 67)

Taking a Few Precautions May Keep You Safe

By trial and error, doctors are gaining ground in the battle to find effective treatments for breast cancer. Ways to prevent the disease are proving more elusive. "We don't know what causes breast cancer, so we don't know how to prevent it," says Dr. Philip Strax, who runs clinics in New York and Florida. Still, medical professionals agree that there are steps you can take to lower your risk. And there are some previously suspect habits—taking a drink or two and using the birth-control pill—that you probably can stop worrying about.

Scientists are not sure how, but a rich diet seems to play a role. Comparisons of breast-cancer rates in other nations have shown a striking relationship between cancer incidence and obesity—the fatter the society, the more women become ill. Women from countries with low-fat diets have a much lower rate of breast cancer than U.S. women do—the rate in Japan, for example, is about one fifth what it is in the U.S.—but the daughters and granddaughters of foreign women who move to the U.S. approach our startling breast-cancer rate of 1 in 10. The death toll among third-generation Japanese American women equals that of other Americans.

Surprisingly, the seemingly obvious defense—to lose weight if you're obese—may not do any good if all you do is cut calories. No one has yet determined whether it's the calories that are the culprit or the same high animal-fat diet that's to blame for so much heart disease. When Wistar Institute scientists in Philadelphia put some rats on high-fat, low-calorie diets and others on low-fat, high-calorie diets, they found that the calories rather than the fat were linked to a greater incidence of cancer. Whether the animal study is relevant to humans is likely to go unanswered. [In January 1988], the National Cancer Institute decided that a planned 10-year, $130 million diet study was just not feasible. And not all research supports a diet-cancer connection. A recent Harvard study of more than 89,000 nurses found no significant association between what women ate and whether they developed breast cancer.

But even without proof, the NCI suggests that women cut fat to no more than 30 percent of a day's total calories. That's because whether obesity or a high-fat diet is to blame, a low-fat diet will offer protection: Lean meats, margarine instead of butter, low-fat dairy products and fewer egg yolks. You may be reducing your breast-cancer risk, and you'll be doing your heart a big favor.

Exercise may help as well. Rose Frisch, a reproductive biologist at Harvard, recently questioned 5,398 college graduates about their health and found the breast-cancer rate among the former athletes was 35 percent less than the rate in more sedentary women. The study didn't determine if it was the exercise itself that made the difference, but Frisch suspects that it was—studies by others in her lab and at Rockefeller University in New York have shown that athletes have lower levels of a form of estrogen that is suspected of playing a role in breast cancer.

Exonerating alcohol

Capping your exercise with a beer shouldn't undo all the benefits, contrary to what Harvard University and National Cancer Institute researchers reported [in 1987]. Their studies indicated that women who took as few as one or two drinks a day were at a higher risk of cancer. Although some smaller studies have hinted before at a connection between alcohol and breast cancer, many scientists found these latest two hard to swallow, because they doubted that such low amounts of alcohol could cause problems. And researchers couldn't explain how alcohol could trigger cancer.

Sure enough, [in 1988] two new studies exonerated alcohol. Susan Chu, an epidemiologist at the Centers for Disease Control in Atlanta, and colleagues questioned about 3,000 women with breast cancer and 3,000 women who did not have cancer about their drinking habits. Her findings—that use of alcohol was unrelated to

WHERE TO GO FOR HELP AND HOPE

CLEARINGHOUSES

■ **American Cancer Society.** Its 3,000 local offices can direct you to local support groups and breast clinics. The ACS also runs its own program, Reach to Recovery, that pairs newly diagnosed women with women who have had breast cancer. For brochures, pamphlets and other information, contact a chapter near you.

■ **National Cancer Institute.** It maintains 26 regional offices, reachable through the Cancer Information Service hot line at (800) 4-CANCER, from 9 a.m. to 10 p.m. Monday through Friday and 10 a.m. to 6 p.m. on Saturday. In Hawaii, it's (808) 524-1234; Hawaiians off Oahu can call collect. Hot-line counselors give answers and will direct you to doctors, hospitals and support groups in your area. For brochures and other information, write to National Cancer Institute, Building 31, Room 10A24, Bethesda, Md. 20892.

REFERRALS

■ **National Cancer Institute,** (800) 4-CANCER.

■ **American Society of Plastic and Reconstructive Surgeons,** (800) 635-0635.

SUPPORT GROUPS

■ **Local hospitals.** Many hospitals, breast clinics and nonprofit organizations maintain breast-cancer support groups. Check your local hospital or ACS office.

■ **ENCORE.** Some YWCA's offer this discussion and exercise program for women who have had breast surgery.

■ **Y-ME,** (800) 221-2141, from 9 a.m. to 5 p.m. central time weekdays, (312) 799-8228 in Chicago and after hours. The line is staffed by counselors who have had breast cancer.

■ **SHARE,** (212) 260-0580. A New York support group for breast-cancer victims.

READING MATERIAL

■ *NABCO News.* The quarterly newsletter of the National Alliance of Breast Cancer Organizations chronicles the latest research and treatment developments in layman's terms. A $25, one-year membership includes a resource list, the newsletter and special mailings. To order, call (212) 719-0154, or write to NABCO, 1180 Avenue of the Americas, New York, N.Y. 10036.

■ *Invisible Scars: A Guide to Coping With the Emotional Impact of Breast Cancer,* Mimi Greenberg, Ph.D., 1988, Walker, New York, N.Y., $17.95.

■ *Alternatives: New Developments in the War on Breast Cancer,* Rose Kushner, 1986, Warner Books, New York, N.Y., $5.95.

■ *Overcoming Breast Cancer,* Genell Subak-Sharpe, 1987, Doubleday, New York, N.Y., $16.95.

■ *Choices: Realistic Alternatives in Cancer Treatment,* Marion Morra and Eve Potts, 1987, Avon Books, New York, N.Y., $10.95.

■ *A Woman's Decision: Breast Care, Treatment and Reconstruction,* Karen Berger and Dr. John Bostwick III, 1988, Quality Medical Publishing, Inc., (800) 423-6865, $12.95.

DETECTION

■ **Mammography.** The American College of Radiology certifies mammography facilities that use special low-dose X-ray machines, have good quality control and trained people on hand. For information on local facilities, call your ACS office or the ACR at (703) 648-8997.

■ **MammaCare.** Write Mammatech Corp., 930 N.W. Eighth Avenue, Gainesville, Fla. 32601, or call (800) MAM-CARE.

---

breast cancer—held true whether one drink a week was consumed or as many as 22 or more. Randall Harris and Dr. Ernst Wynder of the American Health Foundation in New York compared 1,467 women with breast cancer with 10,178 cancer-free women and concluded that while there may be a weak connection, alcohol is not a major factor in breast cancer.

The oral contraceptive pill has also dropped from the list of suspected culprits. Researchers from the Uniformed Services University of the Health Sciences in Bethesda, Md., announced in March [1988] that their study of nearly 5,000 women with breast cancer and 5,000 cancer-free women revealed no association between use of the Pill and breast cancer. On the other hand, since the Pill was only introduced in the early 1960s, it hasn't yet established a long enough track record to get an entirely clean bill of health.

For some women, the prospect of cancer is so horrifying that they prefer to sacrifice the breast in advance rather than live with their fear. Prophylactic mastectomies, or removal of a healthy breast to prevent cancer, should be restricted to women at the very highest risk because of family history, says Dr. William Goodson, director of the breast-screening clinic at the University of California at San Francisco. Goodson feels the operation is appropriate only for women whose risk is 25 percent of higher—women whose mothers or sisters had breast cancer in both breasts after menopause or in one breast before menopause—and even then only if the woman is especially anxious. The surgery was "a small price to pay for peace of mind," says one woman who had a prophylactic mastectomy after watching her mother and grandmother die of breast cancer and undergoing two biopsies herself.

Cancer researchers looking for an option less drastic than surgery are checking out the drug tamoxifen, which robs tumors of the estrogen many need to survive. But this estrogen blocking also causes menopause and may have other side effects when used for a long time. Although some doctors are all for starting a trial now in high-risk older women, others vote for holding off until the long-term effects of tamoxifen are known. A definitive answer is years away.

The best preventions aren't viable. You can't choose to be born into a family whose women are free of breast cancer, and you can't avoid growing old. Since there's no eliminating the risk, the key is to first minimize it, and then keep an eagle eye out for the danger signs.

Source: Joanne Silberner, *U.S. News and World Report* (11 July 1988), pp. 60–61.

35 and 40 receive a baseline examination. Follow-up examinations every 1 to 2 years between the ages of 40 and 49 are recommended. For women aged 50 and older, annual checkups are in order.

3. Health practitioner examinations periodically, once every 3 years between the ages of 20 and 40, annually for those over age 40.

Each of these steps is necessary to detect breast cancer early. Each element alone is not accurate enough to exclude use of the other methods of screening. Many women complain that they aren't sure what they are feeling for when they do a breast self-examination. It takes time to learn what normal breast tissue feels like. But doing the examination several times will help acquaint a woman with what is normal for her. Doctors recommend that each woman do the examination on the last day of the

FIGURE 3.4
Breast Self-Examination

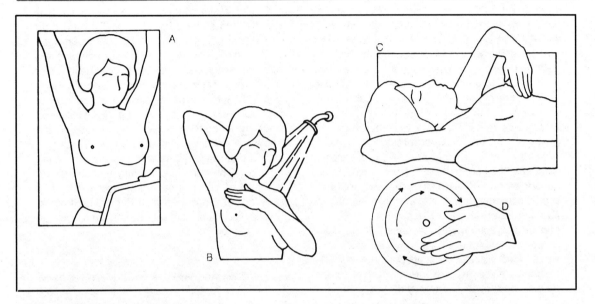

Source: the American Cancer Society.

It is important for a woman to examine her breasts regularly. She should look at her breasts in the mirror, first with her arms at her sides, then with them raised over her head (A). Visible warning signals include thickening, swelling, dimpling, skin irritation, distortion, retraction, or scaliness. In the shower, her hands can easily move over the wet skin (B). When she is lying down a woman can easily examine her breast tissue as it is distributed (C). The fingers should be held flat and move in complete clockwise circles around the outer portion of the breast, then move progressively inward toward the nipple (D). Warning signals that can be detected include a lump or lumps, thickening, pain or tenderness of the nipple, or discharge.

menstrual period, a time when the breasts are least likely to be tender and swollen from the effects of hormones, and a time that is easy to remember. Post-menopausal women may choose the beginning or end of the calendar month to remind them to do the examination regularly. In general, those tumors found by BSE are smaller than those found in women who do not do BSE. [15] Tumors must be at least 1 centimeter in size to be felt by physical examination.

The purpose of mammography is to find cancers before they can be felt during a self-examination. Mammography is a mildly uncomfortable X-ray procedure that involves placing the breast between 2 plates, applying gentle pressure to flatten the breast, then taking an X ray with a very small amount of radiation exposure. Periodic mammography screenings can lessen one's chances of dying from breast cancer by as much as 20 to 30 percent. The greatest advantage occurs in women over age 50, but the procedure also benefits women under 50. [16] The risk of developing cancer from the radiation exposure associated with mammography is 1 in every 1 million women exposed. Since the statistical risk of breast cancer is 1 in 10, the risk associated with the procedure is greatly outweighed by the potential benefit.

Cancer of the Colon and Rectum

The colon and rectum are at the end of the digestive tract. The colon, also called the large intestine or bowel, functions to extract water from the already-digested food. It then holds this solid waste matter until it is eliminated from the body.

The American Cancer Society estimates there were 155,000 new cases of cancer of the colon and rectum in 1990. [17] This cancer is the second most common cause of cancer death. The term "colorectal cancer" refers to these two cancers combined. According to the American Cancer Society, "When detected early and treated promptly, over three-quarters of all such patients can be cured and are able to return to work." [18]

Signs and Symptoms Colorectal cancer has a wide range of symptoms, including diarrhea, constipation, or both alternately. Bleeding, narrowing of the stool, an increase in abdominal discomfort or gas, or a sensation that the bowel never empties may be signs of colon or rectal cancer. If any of the symptoms are present, seek medical attention.

As with other forms of cancer, a biopsy is necessary to make a diagnosis. Often, if the symptoms suggest a cancer, an X ray of the colon, called a **barium enema**, will be necessary. A direct viewing of the rectum and colon by **proctosigmoidoscopy** may also be recommended. Proctosigmoidoscopy is a procedure that involves inserting a scoping instrument into the patient's rectum to allow the examining physician to view directly the lining of the bowel. Newer, flexible instruments for this procedure provide a significant improvement in comfort compared to the older, rigid scopes. [19] Depending on the length of the bowel that needs to be viewed, either a flexible **sigmoidoscopy** or a **colonoscopy** is done. As a screening procedure, a sigmoidoscopy that views the last 50 centimeters of the colon (called the sigmoid colon because it forms the shape of an S-curve) is done. A colonoscopy, which views the entire colon, is recommended for those with known

(continued on p. 71)

Barium enema: A process in which barium sulfate, a chemical that is visible on X rays, is introduced into the bowel so that the lining of the colon and rectum can be examined by X ray.

Proctosigmoidoscopy: A procedure that involves the visual inspection of the lower (sigmoid) colon and rectum via a viewing instrument known as a proctosigmoidoscope.

Sigmoidoscopy: A screening procedure that involves viewing the last 50 centimeters of the colon (called the sigmoid colon because it forms the shape of an S-curve) with a short, flexible, viewing device called a sigmoidoscope.

Colonoscopy: A procedure that involves viewing the inside of the entire colon, usually for diagnostic purposes, by means of a long, flexible instrument called a colonoscope.

Although the word polyp comes from the Latin *polypus,* meaning "many-footed" (like an octopus), in English the word has evolved to mean something protruding from a flat surface. Polyps develop from many of the tissues that form lining surfaces in the body, but they are especially common in the large intestine.

Most bowel cancers originate in polyps, and the precancerous, or

The Various Kinds of Polyp

adenomatous, type (also called *adenomas*) increase in prevalence after age 50. At any one time, the vast majority of polyps are benign, and cancer develops slowly in them, probably over the course of many years.

Four important characteristics are used to estimate the cancerous potential of an adenomatous polyp: its size; whether or not it has a stalk; the microscopic organization of cells within it; and the microscopic appearance of the cells themselves.

- Larger polyps (over a centimeter in diameter) are more likely to develop cancer.
- Polyps with a stalk (*pedunculated*) are less threatening than those sitting directly on the bowel wall (*sessile*), if for no other reason than that cancer originating in the head of a pedunculated polyp has further to travel before it can spread to and beyond the bowel wall.
- Broadly speaking, cells within a polyp may be organized according to either of two major patterns. In *tubular* polyps, cells form microscopic tube-like structures. This is the less ominous pattern; fewer than 2% of these polyps contain cancer when found by colonoscopy. In *villous adenomas,* the cells form fronds rather than tubules. About one-fifth of villous adenomas already contain cancer when they are discovered by colonoscopy (but malignant tissue may not be included in a snippet of tissue taken for biopsy). *Tubulovillous adenomas* contain elements of both growth patterns; the villous component is the more worrisome.
- Whether a polyp can be called benign, precancerous, or cancerous depends on the individual cells within it. As cells progress toward the malignant state, features within them become distorted. This process of distortion is called *dysplasia* until it reaches a stage that is frankly cancerous. A cancer is called *carcinoma in situ* until it begins to invade the bowel wall. At this point it is termed *invasive cancer.* Once cancer has traveled to distant locations, such as lymph nodes or the liver, it is called *metastatic.*

Villous adenomas are virtually always sessile and are the type most likely to become cancerous. So a villous adenoma should be removed. It may be cauterized (*fulgurated*) through a flexible sigmoidoscope or may require surgery for removal. Tubular adenomas usually pose a smaller risk.

Many polyps found in the intestine have no malignant potential. In some families, however, the inherited tendency to develop multiple polyps is a sign of high risk for cancer. At the extreme, *familial polyposis* of the colon, in which the bowel lining may be studded with thousands of polyps, carries a 100% risk that a malignancy will develop by early adulthood. Removal of the colon is always recommended for these people.

Source: *Harvard Medical School Health Letter,* Vol. 14, No. 11, September 1989, pp. 2–3.

polyps. Polyps are abnormal growths of tissue in the lining of the bowel that protrude into the canal of the intestine. If a polyp is found, a piece of the tissue can be taken at the time of scoping or the entire polyp may be removed. A biopsy is then performed on the growth.

Early diagnosis of colon and rectal cancer greatly improves the chances for cure and long-term survival. Those whose colon cancer is detected while still localized have nearly a 90 percent 5-year survival rate. Rectal cancer victims have a 5-year survival rate of nearly 80 percent when it is found in a localized stage. Treatment of colorectal cancer almost always involves surgery and is cured in 45 to 50 percent of cases. [20] Radiation is also commonly used in rectal cancer. Chemotherapy may be used in either.

Recommendations for Periodic Screening   Although some controversy exists over their efficacy, 3 easy screening tests have been recommended by the American Cancer Society to detect colorectal cancer:

1. *Digital rectal examination:* This may be done annually after the age of 40. A physician inserts a gloved finger into the rectum and feels the lining of the rectum. In men, examination of the prostate is done at the same time.

2. *Stool blood test:* Recommended as a yearly test after the age of 50, it involves taking a small amount of stool from each of 3 consecutive bowel movements and mounting it on a prepared slide. The slide is returned to the medical practitioner's office and tested for the presence of blood.

3. *Proctosigmoidoscopy:* Sometimes called a "procto." This is a screening procedure recommended for those over 50. The first

FIGURE 3.5
Polyps in the Intestinal Wall

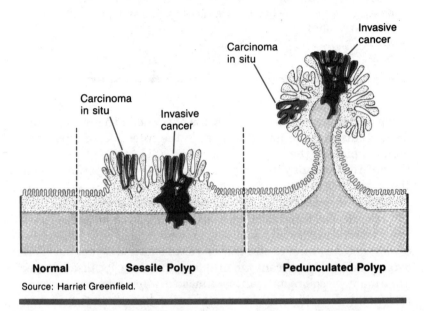

Carcinoma in situ

Invasive cancer

Carcinoma in situ

Invasive cancer

Normal   **Sessile Polyp**   **Pedunculated Polyp**

Source: Harriet Greenfield.

A section of intestinal wall is illustrated. Two kinds of polyp protrude into the interior of the large bowel. Both are cancerous.

test is usually followed up by a second within a 12-month period. If both tests are normal, subsequent examinations may be needed only every 3 to 5 years.

Risk Factors   The cause of colon cancer is unknown, but a few risk factors have been identified. The presence of a polyp increases the risk of colon cancer. The larger the polyp, the more likely that it is cancerous. Colorectal cancer rates may be reduced if polyps are detected early and removed before they become cancerous. Someone with a family history of colorectal cancer should pay particular attention to this as a cause of cancer. For example, there are a few inherited forms of polyps, called familial polyposis, which are known to increase the risk of colon cancer. If a person has a history of inflammatory bowel disease (ulcerative colitis or Crohn's disease), he or she is also at increased risk of developing colorectal cancer.

Newer studies are implicating diet as a risk factor for colon cancer. A diet that is high in fat and low in fiber, with insufficient grains and fresh fruit, may be a causative factor.

Uterine Cancer

Uterine cancer is the fourth most common cancer diagnosed in women. However, the death rate from this cancer has declined 70 percent over the past 40 years. This is no doubt primarily because of both the Pap smear test and regular checkups. [21]

There are two locations for uterine cancer, the **uterine cervix** and the **endometrium**. Of the estimated 46,500 cases of uterine cancer in 1990, 13,500 cases will be cervical and 33,000 cases will involve the endometrium, or the lining of the uterus. [22]

Signs and Symptoms   Often (until late in the course of the disease) there are no signs or symptoms of cervical cancer. However, if bleeding occurs between menstrual periods or after menopause, or if an unusual vaginal discharge is present, a prompt medical evaluation is recommended.

Diagnosis and Treatment   Diagnosis usually begins with the **Pap smear**. This test involves obtaining a sample of cells by scraping the cervix with a small spatula or swab. The cells are transferred to a slide to be viewed under a microscope. If abnormal cells are detected, a biopsy is taken. The Pap test is best suited for detecting cancer of the cervix but only partially effective in detecting endometrial cancer. Women, especially those over 40, with abnormal bleeding may need an endometrial sampling.

Treatment of cervical and endometrial cancer involves surgery, radiation, or a combination of both. In precancerous stages, cervical growths may be treated with freezing (cryotherapy), by destroying tissue with heat by electric current (electrocoagulation), or with local surgery. Precancerous changes associated with endometrial cancer have been treated with progesterone hormone, but the success rate is debated.

Recommendations for Periodic Screening   Every woman over age 18 should undergo a Pap test and pelvic exam annually until 3 consecutive examinations have been normal. Then tests may be repeated less frequently at the discretion of the medical practitioner. Women at risk for endometrial cancer should have endometrial tissue sampling done around the time of menopause.

Uterine cervix: The neck of the uterus, which protrudes into the top of the vaginal canal.

Endometrium: The lining of the uterus.

Pap smear: A test designed to detect abnormal changes in a small smple containing cells from the surface of the cervix (the neck of the uterus).

FIGURE 3.6
Pap Test Evaluation

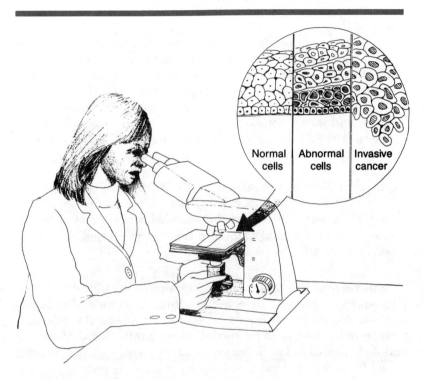

Source: American College of Obstetricians and Gynecologists.

The magnified detail shows normal cervical cells, a layer of abnormal cells growing up toward the surface of the cervix, and invasive cancer cells. A Pap test can help detect changes in the cervix before cancer develops, when cure rates are highest.

Risk Factors   The risk factors for cancer at the two sites differ. For cervical cancer, the risk factors are first intercourse at an early age, multiple sexual partners, contracting certain sexually transmitted diseases, and cigarette smoking. [23] Diagnosis of uterine cancer is usually made after the age of 50. Risk factors include having never borne children, a failure to ovulate, obesity, and prolonged estrogen therapy.

Estrogen and Uterine Cancer   For many years, estrogen has been prescribed for women to treat symptoms of menopause. More recently, estrogen therapy has been used in the hope of protecting women from the problems of osteoporosis, the increased bone loss that occurs during menopause. If estrogen levels are kept normal, bone loss is diminished. However, it has now been shown that prolonged use of estrogen, uninterrupted by progesterone, can lead to endometrial cancer. The use of postmenopausal estrogen in women who have not had a hysterectomy may include the use of progesterone to diminish the risk of developing uterine cancer.

Cancer of the Prostate and Testes

Cancer of the prostate is third only to lung cancer and cancer of the colon and rectum as the most common cancer in men. It is rare before age 50; 80 percent of the diagnosed cases occur in men aged 65 and older. Particularly at risk are men living in North America and Europe. For reasons that are not yet known, it is more common among black males than among white males in the United States. [24]

Warning signs include a weak or interrupted flow of urine; inability to urinate; difficulty starting or stopping the flow of urine; frequency of urination, especially at night; blood in the urine; or pain in the lower back or thighs.

Because the cause of prostate cancer is unknown, there are no known actions to prevent its occurrence. Early detection and prompt treatment are the only known defenses. Screening for prostate cancer involves a digital rectal examination by your health-care professional. This examination is recommended annually for men over the age of 40. When prostate cancer is suspected, a biopsy of prostate tissue is performed.

Treatment of prostatic cancer may include surgical removal of the prostate gland and exploration of the surrounding tissues and lymph nodes. Impotence frequently accompanies this radical surgery, but urinary incontinence rarely occurs. Limited prostate cancer requires less radical surgery. Radiation has also been used in treating prostate cancer, in the hope of maintaining potency while ridding the affected area(s) of cancer.

Growth of normal prostate tissue depends on the presence of male hormones. Depriving the body of these hormones by castration (the surgical removal of the testicles) or adding female hormone (estrogen) has long been shown to decrease the bone pain associated with prostate cancer metastases. Bone is the most common site of metastasis for prostate cancer. [25]

Cancer of the testes is not very common but is mentioned for 3 reasons. First, testicular carcinoma is most common among young men, those between the ages of 20 and 35. Second, a

(continued on p. 77)

A Costly Sense of Squeamishness

A comparison of prostate cancer and breast cancer turns up intriguing parallels. Prostate cancer will strike 1 in 11 men at some point in their lives; breast cancer will strike 1 in 10 women. Both are cancers of the reproductive tissue, and both kill tens of thousands of Americans a year, many of them people who could have lived if their disease had been detected early.

The connection with sex makes both cancers a subject of discomfiture, but there the similarity ends. Women clearly have less trouble thinking and talking about breast cancer than men do about prostate cancer. When was the last time a male celebrity discussed his prostate cancer on the TV-talk-show circuit? How many men have written autobiographies dealing with the effect the cancer had on their lives? "There has been no male Betty Ford or Ann Jillian or Gloria Steinem," says Rose Kushner, an advocate for women with breast cancer who had the disease herself. For reasons seemingly rooted in psychology, women have brought breast cancer out in the open over the past 15 years, while men have kept prostate cancer locked up in their psychic closets.

The silence has dire consequences. Without public discussion, prostate cancer gets only a trickle of federal research funding, delaying the arrival of better ways to diagnose and treat the disease. Meanwhile, breast-cancer patients can tap into myriad support groups aimed at women who share their problems. There is only one advocacy group for men with prostate cancer, called Patient Advocates for Advanced Cancer Treatments (PAACT, 1143 Parmelee, N.W., Grand Rapids, Mich. 49504. Call 616-453-1477). PAACT, with fewer than 4,000 members, runs support groups and is a clearinghouse for information about various investigational treatments, though it is more enthusiastic about some of these treatments than experts say is warranted.

The only other support groups are those run by the American Cancer Society and organizations aimed at people with various kinds of cancer rather than one particular disease. Many men do not feel comfortable talking in such open settings about incontinence and impotence that sometimes arise from treatment. "So they're walking around in diapers, they're impotent, with penile implants, and they don't want to talk about it," says Kushner. "And they're not going to go to a legislature and try to raise funds."

Perhaps the most insidious ripple to spread from such self-consciousness is this: Because men with prostate cancer rarely proselytize about early detection and treatment, the same fate unnecessarily befalls some of their confreres. Women with breast cancer can teach men much, if men are willing to learn.

Prostate vs. breast cancer

The projected number of new cases and deaths in 1989 for prostate and breast cancer are roughly similar. The federal funds spent in fiscal 1989 on research and education are not.

	Prostate cancer	Breast cancer
Cases	103,000	142,900
Deaths	28,500	43,300
Federal funding	$9.5 mil.	$70.8 mil.

USN&WR--Basic data: American Cancer Society, National Cancer Institute

Source: Joanne Silberner, *U.S. News and World Report* (10 July 1989), pp. 56–57.

FIGURE 3.7
Testicular Self-Examination

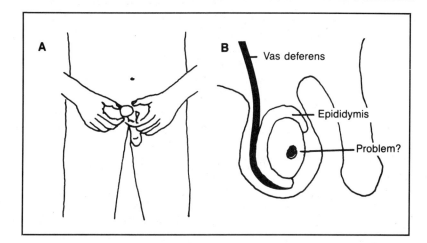

Source: American Cancer Society.

The best time for a man to examine his testes is right after a hot bath or shower because the testicle descends and the scrotal skin relaxes in the heat. He should place his index and middle fingers on the underside of the testicle and his thumbs on top (A). He should gently roll the testicle between his fingers and thumb. Any abnormal lump is most likely to be found at the front or side of the testicle (B).

regular self-examination may detect it early (each testicle should be gently rolled between the thumb and finger to check for evidence of any nodules or hard lumps). Third, if found in its early stages, testicular cancer is curable. A man who finds a lump in either of his testicles should see his physician immediately.

Leukemia and Lymphomas
Leukemia refers to a group of cancers of the blood-forming cells that proliferate in bone marrow and lymph tissues. These abnormal cells interfere with the normal production of cells that help fight off infection, cells that help blood to clot, and red cells, which carry oxygen to the organs. Symptoms of leukemia include frequent infections, fever, easy bruising, and the fatigue associated with anemia.

There are two patterns to leukemia: acute and chronic. The acute form comes on rapidly. Its symptoms, fever or bruising and

Hodgkin's disease: A cancer of the lymph tissue (lymph nodes, spleen) in which the malignant cells reproduce rapidly and cause a swelling of the lymph nodes, typically those in the neck or armpits.

Basal cell cancer (carcinoma): The most common and least dangerous form of skin cancer; basal cell cancers originate in the basal layer of the skin; they grow slowly and seldom spread to other areas of the body.

Squamous cell cancer (carcinoma): A form of skin cancer that usually takes the form of red, scaly patches or lesions on the lips, face, or tips of the ears; if left untreated, squamous cell cancers can spread to other parts of the body.

Melanoma: A skin cancer derived from the pigment-secreting cells in the skin; it is highly malignant and may cause death.

lymph node enlargement, are easy to recognize. Quick treatment of the acute form is essential or death will occur within months. [26] Even with treatment, there is only a 34 percent 5-year survival rate. [27] The chronic form may have any of the same symptoms or no symptoms at all. Adults, with approximately 25,000 cases a year, are more likely to be affected than children. Even so, 2,500 children contract leukemia each year.

The cause of leukemia in most patients is not known, but experts believe that both genetic susceptibility and environmental factors play a role. Leukemia affects both sexes and all ages. Specific types of leukemia have been linked to excessive radiation exposure: "Japanese survivors of the atomic bomb explosions have a predictable and dose-related increased incidence of leukemia." [28] Exposure to certain chemicals, such as benzene, is also linked to leukemia. Only one kind of leukemia is known to be caused by a virus.

Lymphomas are a group of malignant conditions arising from the lymph tissues. The symptoms of these cancers are related to impaired immunity. **Hodgkin's disease** accounts for about 40 percent of these cancers. The incidence of lymphoma has been increasing each year, but deaths have been decreasing as a result of improved treatment. Having painless but enlarged lymph nodes is the most common symptom of the disease, although fever, night sweats, or fatigue may also occur. The cause of lymphoma is not yet known. As with leukemia, genetics, environmental factors, and even viruses are suspected in its development.

Leukemias and lymphomas differ from the other common forms of cancer discussed in this book because periodic screening and prevention, except with regard to X ray and benzene avoidance, have not shown to be beneficial to survival.

Skin Cancers

Skin cancers are the most common form of cancer. There are more than 600,000 cases reported each year. The most common form of skin cancer—about 75 percent of all cases—is **basal cell cancer,** which is highly treatable. **Squamous cell cancers** are a more serious—but also treatable—form of skin cancer. **Melanoma** is the most dangerous skin cancer. Incidence is growing at the rate of 4 percent a year. [29] Although melanoma accounted for only 5 percent of all skin cancers in 1990, it was responsible for 75 percent of the deaths from skin cancers. What makes melanoma so deadly is that it is more likely than other skin cancers to metastasize to other parts of the body. Early recognition and treatment of melanoma is the best defense against its fatal effects.

(continued on p. 81)

The Melanoma Epidemic

Malignant melanoma, according to new statistics, could become a lethal epidemic in the next decade. More people are getting melanoma, a cancer of the pigmented skin cells, and they are getting it when they are younger. Cancer researchers, the American Academy of Dermatology, and the American Cancer Society (ACS) are publicizing the need for prevention and for early detection, which is crucial for cure.

[In 1990 an estimated], 27,600 people in the [U.S. developed melanoma], and 6,300 [died] from it. One in 120 Americans can expect to develop this cancer during his or her lifetime—a twelvefold increase since the 1930s, when the figure was only 1 in 1,500.

Exactly *why* the rate of skin cancer is growing so rapidly is not known. Although depletion of the ozone in the stratosphere will increase the rate of squamous- and basal-cell skin cancers, its effect on melanoma is unclear.

New evidence implicates sun-worship, which burgeoned during the 1950s and 1960s, especially among teenagers. The bronzed youth of the baby boom, now reaching middle age, are in the vanguard of the melanoma plague.

"What is most startling about these numbers is that the greatest rate of increase is in people under the age of 40, and particularly women under the age of 40," says Dr. Darrell S. Rigel, a dermatologist at New York University Medical Center.

Blistering sunburns suffered during childhood and adolescence, according to Dr. Rigel, are now believed to be the trigger for melanoma, which then takes 20–30 years to develop. "It appears in certain new studies that the risk of melanoma is particularly related to the duration and intensity of sun exposure received during the teen years. If you had three or more blistering sunburns before the age of about 20, the risk of developing melanoma is four to five times that of someone who had no blistering sunburns."

In comparing melanoma patients with similar people free of the disease, Dr. Arthur Sober of the Melanoma Research Unit at Massachusetts General Hospital and his colleagues found that the major risk factors were traceable to childhood and adolescence; they were blistering from sunburns, getting a tan only with difficulty, and being taken to warm, sunny places for extended vacations. Recent studies conducted at New York University show that people who worked outdoors for three or more years as teenagers have triple the average risk for melanoma.

Sunburn is the key influence leading to an increase in melanoma, but *who* gets the disease is also determined by heredity. About 10% of all cases run in families. Because they are at very high risk of developing the malignancy, people with a family history of melanoma should practice frequent self-examination of their skin and make regular visits to a personal physician or dermatologist for checkups and, if necessary, early treatment.

Several other risk factors have been identified. People with fair skin, blond or red hair, or marked freckling of the upper back are more likely to get melanoma. Also at increased risk are people who have actinic keratoses, usually developing after age 40. These are small, slightly scaly bumps (often more easily felt than seen) that are the color of surrounding skin or somewhat darker; they indicate cumulative exposure to sunlight. Merely living close to the equator, which increases exposure to ultraviolet light, may be a predisposing factor. In 1978–81, the last time the ACS collected such statistics, Atlanta's melanoma rate was 11 cases per 100,000 residents, while Detroit's was 6 per 100,000. Tucson, with more sunny days than Atlanta, has the highest reported rate in the United States, 27 per 100,000.

Total sun exposure over one's lifetime should be factored into the overall estimate of risk, according to Dr. Carl Washington, a dermatologic surgeon at Emory Clinic in Atlanta. "Every exposure to ultraviolet rays is stored in our skin. Unlike tans, which fade in the winter, the damage done by ultraviolet exposure is cumulative." Although dark skin is less vulnerable to melanoma and other skin cancers, Dr. Washington points out that "it is still possible for blacks and deep-toned people to develop melanoma on the palms of the hands, on the soles of the feet, and even in the mouth"—although probably not as a result of sun exposure. In 1986 the reported rate of melanoma among blacks was about one-fiftieth of that among whites.

Damage control

Preventing melanoma is a long-term project that requires shielding youngsters from sunlight. Dr. Robert Stern, a dermatologist at Boston's Beth Israel Hospital, and his colleagues have estimated that if everyone below the age of 18 regularly used a sunscreen with a sun protective factor of 15, the lifetime incidence of nonmelanoma skin cancers (basal cell and squamous cell) would be reduced by three-quarters. It seems probable that the risk of melanomas would also decline.

Parents should begin regularly applying sunscreen to their toddlers and educating them about the hazards of overexposure. As Dr. Mary Spraker, a dermatologist at Emory University who specializes in the skin diseases of children, says: "A tan is not beautiful. A tan means damage." Dr. Spraker advises parents to get tough and stay tough about sun exposure—for the entire summer. "All children should wear hats and stay out of the sun between 11 A.M. and 2 P.M. During the late spring and summer, children should not be sent out to play at noontime, when the sun is strongest."

The hardest part may be convincing teenagers—who believe they are immortal—that their age group is at high risk. But Dr. Spraker says she is seeing some encouraging signs that Americans' love affair with the tan is waning. "More and more, women's magazines are printing interviews with models who say they use sunscreens or avoid sun exposure altogether. Some ads for bathing suits in . . . magazines are showing untanned models. And a new airline travel billboard features a woman in a bathing suit, sitting on the beach, but under an umbrella."

For mad dogs, Englishmen, and other people who have already spent too much time in the midday sun, melanoma can no longer be prevented, but early detection can permit curative removal. The ACS proposes that all people, especially those at high risk, perform skin self-examinations, like breast or testicular exams, every month. The object is to spot potentially malignant lesions. The entire skin surface should be inspected, with the aid of mirrors, for any change in the size, texture, or color of a pigmented area, for visible spots that are oozing fluid, bleeding easily, or newly itchy, and for moles that meet the "ABCD" criteria (*see below*).

If self-inspection turns up any suspicious skin changes, a prompt visit to one's family physician is indicated, according to the ACS, because early removal of a melanoma is the *only* factor making a significant difference in survival statistics for this fast-spreading cancer.

Sunscreens

Is a sun protective factor (SPF) of 15 just as good as SPF 30? Perhaps not. For most people, both preparations will prevent reddening from a day in the sun. (The SPF is assigned on the basis of its ability to prevent reddening after measured exposure to intense, artificial ultraviolet light.) But redness is not the only effect of sun damage. Microscopic changes (which cannot be detected without a skin biopsy) appear even when sunburn has been prevented, according to dermatologist Kays H. Kaidbey at the University of Pennsylvania, reporting in the March [1990] *Journal of the American Academy of Dermatology*. SPF 30 is more effective than SPF 15 in reducing these microscopic changes.

Currently, products with SPF 15 or more are recommended for general use. A higher rating is recommended for anyone who still burns despite applying a preparation rated at 15. Products labeled "waterproof" offer protection in the water for about 80 minutes, whereas those designated "water resistant" are only good for about 40 minutes.

The product, whether a gel, a lotion, or an ointment, should be applied to the skin about 15 minutes before exposure to the sun. This interval permits the active ingredients to become more firmly attached to the skin. Sunscreen should be reapplied every 60–90 minutes, especially if perspiration is heavy.

The ABCD Rule

What is the difference between an ordinary mole and a life-threatening melanoma?

Asymmetry: Most moles are symmetrical. If you drew a line through the middle, the two halves would mirror each other. Melanomas are asymmetric; their two halves are not mirror images.

Border: Most moles have a distinct border. The border of a melanoma is likely to be notched, scalloped, or indistinct.

Color: Moles may be either dark or light, but they tend to be all the same color. Early melanomas are likely to be uneven in color or a mixture of several different hues.

Diameter: Once a melanoma has acquired its A, B, and C characteristics, it is also likely to be more than 6 millimeters wide (about the diameter of a pencil eraser).

Source: *Harvard Medical School Health Letter,* Vol. 15, No. 8, June 1990, pp. 1–3.

Causes and Prevention The sun's ultraviolet rays cause skin cancers. These rays are strongest between the hours of 10 A.M. and 3 P.M., so exposure during this time should be avoided. Anytime you are in sunlight, you should wear protective clothing and a hat and use ointment sunscreens. The lower-ranked sunscreens, with ratings of from 1 to 8, offer little protection against sunburn. Instead, use the higher-ranked sunscreens, 8 to 15 or higher. Severe sunburn during childhood has been linked to melanoma later in life, making it especially important to protect children from traumatic sunburn. [30] For those with prolonged sun exposure, such as lifeguards, people who fish for a living, and the like, zinc oxide, an opaque sunscreen, is recommended. It can be used to cover exposed vulnerable areas, such as the nose and lips.

Signs and Symptoms Areas of the body exposed to the sun are the most likely places for basal cell and squamous cell cancers to occur. These include the face, neck, forearms, and the back of the hands. Cancerous areas often appear pearly or waxy, but skin cancer may also take the form of unhealing sores. Because they are slow-growing and rarely metastasize, they are usually curable.

A melanoma, on the other hand, often appears as a change in the size, color, or shape of an existing mole, or as a new mole-like growth that rapidly increases in size. It is usually black or dark brown and may have irregular or uneven borders. Although a melanoma can occur anywhere, its usual locations are on the trunk, head, neck, arm, or leg.

Did You Know That . . .

The ozone layer in the Earth's atmosphere screens out harmful ultraviolet radiation. Experts estimate that, if the ozone layer continues to deteriorate at its current rate, there will be 12 million new cases of skin cancer in the United States over the next 50 years, causing 200,000 deaths.

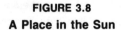

FIGURE 3.8
A Place in the Sun

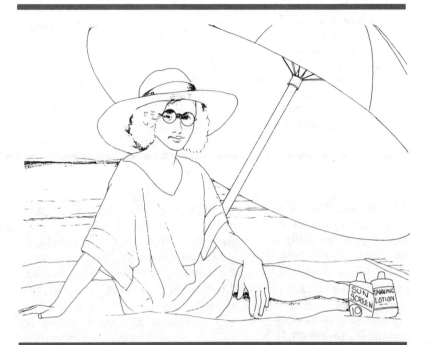

Wearing protective clothing when going out in the sun, using a sunscreen with a protective factor of 15 or greater, and avoiding the sun's rays at the peak hours from 10 A.M. to 3 P.M. will reduce your risk of skin cancer.

Diagnosis and Treatment   The diagnosis of skin cancer usually results from a biopsy of tissue from the suspicious area. Although several different treatments are acceptable for squamous and basal cell cancers, surgery is necessary to treat malignant melanoma. The initial treatment for melanoma is surgical removal of the tumor and all skin surrounding it to a 5-centimeter radius, a procedure that often requires skin grafts. Doctors will then dissect the nearby lymph nodes to determine whether the tumor has metastasized. This dissection may also decrease the total number of cancer cells. Metastasis may occur anywhere, but the brain and liver are common sites. Once the cancer has spread, death usually occurs within a year. [31] The 5-year survival rate for nonmetastasized malignant melanoma is 81 percent. For other skin cancers, it is 95 percent. [32] Early detection is absolutely critical for melanoma because it metastasizes early.

Everyone should perform skin self-examinations every month, regardless of age. Although other skin cancers rarely occur in a child, melanomas can occur at any age.

Risk Factors   Excessive exposure to the sun's ultraviolet rays is the most common cause of skin cancer, especially among fair-skinned people. Other risk factors include occupational exposures to coal tar, pitch, creosote, arsenic compounds, or radium. Skin cancers rarely occur in blacks because of their heavier skin pigmentation. [33]

CLOSING OBSERVATIONS ON PREVENTING CANCER

The cause of cancer is an equation with several terms. First add together or multiply the risk factors, then subtract preventive measures. To increase the odds that this equation will turn out in your favor, diminish the risk factors, enhance the preventive measures, get periodic screenings for cancer, and keep a watchful eye for signs and symptoms.

Risk factors vary according to the form of cancer. Overall, the best way to lessen the risk factors is to reduce or eliminate dangerous life-style practices. Here are the most important steps you can take:

1. *Quit smoking.* Cigarette smoking is the single biggest cancer risk factor of all and causes 30 percent of all cancers.

2. *Lower the fat content in your diet.* High fat diets have been linked with breast, prostate, and colon cancers. Eat leaner meats, fish, skinned poultry, and low-fat dairy products.

3. *Consume alcohol in moderation*—the equivalent of less than 2 ounces of hard liquor, 8 ounces of wine, or 24 ounces of beer a day. Excessive alcohol comsumption increases the risk of cancer, especially when combined with smoking.

4. *Avoid salt-cured, smoked, or nitrite-cured foods.* These may increase the risk of cancers of the esophagus and stomach. If you eat such foods, do so only occasionally.

Occupational risk factors, such as exposure to radiation or radon, and the risk posed by estrogen intake are factors that

Did You Know That . . .

From 1973 to 1985 the mortality rate for skin cancer in the United States increased 25.9 percent.

should be considered on a case-by-case basis. Individual self-education is important here, so information regarding these issues may be obtained from your local chapter of the American Cancer Society or from your health-care provider.

Where diet is concerned, the cabbage family of vegetables— broccoli, cauliflower, Brussels sprouts, cabbage, and kale— appears to protect against colorectal, stomach, and respiratory cancers. Experts believe that a high-fiber diet helps protect against colon cancer. The best natural sources of fiber are grains such as wheat and bran cereals, rice, popcorn, and whole-grain breads; fruits, including peaches and strawberries; and vegetables such as potatoes, spinach, and tomatoes. Foods high in vitamin A may offer protection against the risk of cancers of the esophagus, larynx, and lung. Fruits such as peaches and apricots, and vegetables such as carrots, squash, and broccoli are good sources of vitamin A. Another vitamin natural to fruits and vegetables, vitamin C, may protect against cancers of the esophagus and stomach. Citrus fruits, cantaloupe, red and green peppers, broccoli, and tomatoes are all good sources of vitamin C.

On a related topic, obesity is linked to several cancers, including cancer of the uterus, gallbladder, breast, and colon. Weight reduction, therefore, may decrease the risk of certain cancers. [34]

For protection against skin cancers, include these 3 steps:

1. Avoid exposure to the sun's rays when they are most intense, between 10 A.M. and 3 P.M..

2. Wear protective clothing, such as long sleeves, long pants or skirts, and hats.

3. Use sunscreens rated at levels 8 to 15 or above.

Personal surveillance for any of the warning signs of cancer should be an ongoing concern. Monthly breast self-examination is recommended for all women. Men should do a monthly exam of their testicles. Members of both sexes should also examine themselves for signs of skin cancer each month. A cancer-related checkup has been recommended by the American Cancer Society. Its guidelines suggest such an examination every 3 years between the ages of 20 and 40, and annually after the age of 40. It includes both a physical examination and health counseling.

Experts are making advances in the diagnosis and treatment of cancer daily. Still, prevention and early detection remain the best available methods to combat this deadly disease. ▨

Diseases of the Lung

L UNG DISEASE—excluding lung cancer—is the fifth most common cause of death in the United States. It is the third most common reason for disability benefits. [1] Experts estimate that 20 percent of all adult men have some form of lung disease. Cigarette smoking accounted for approximately 85 percent of the 60,000 deaths from lung disease in 1983. [2]

The two most common chronic lung diseases in adults are chronic bronchitis and emphysema, but other conditions, such as occupational lung diseases, asthma, and general infections, are also hazardous. How these diseases are treated and prevented is the focus of this chapter.

THE STRUCTURE AND FUNCTION OF THE LUNGS

The lungs are part of the respiratory system. The components that comprise this part of the body are the nasal cavity; the throat; the larynx, or voice box; the windpipe; the bronchi; and the lungs. All of these elements are involved in the act of breathing. Breathing is the process whereby the lungs draw in air and its vital oxygen and then expel air as carbon dioxide.

The primary function of the lungs is to facilitate this exchange of gases. These organs extract oxygen from the air we breathe in and release carbon dioxide, a waste-product of metabolism, to be exhaled. The structure of the lung fits its purpose well. The **trachea**, or windpipe, resembles the trunk of a tree, which branches off into several smaller airways called **bronchi** and **bronchioles**. The airways terminate in air sacs called **alveoli**.

Trachea: The windpipe that connects the airways of the lungs to the mouth.

Bronchi: The two large tubular airways that connect the air sacs of the lung with the trachea.

Bronchioles: The smallest airways within the lungs that connect the air sacs of the lung with the bronchi.

Alveoli: The small air sacs of the lung, where the blood exchanges carbon dioxide for oxygen.

The human lungs are complex biological pumps that draw in and push out 10,000 to 12,000 quarts of air each day.

FIGURE 4.1
The Respiratory System

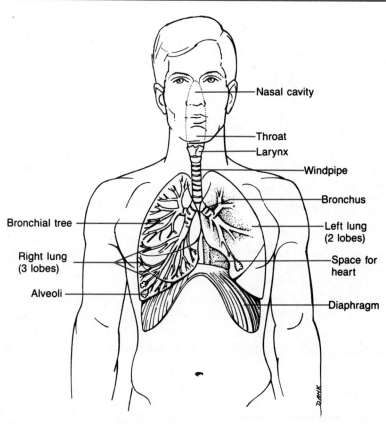

Source: Leonard Dank, Medical Illustrations.

This diagram shows the major components of the respiratory system.

Chronic bronchitis: A persistent inflammation of the bronchial tubes accompanied by the coughing up of excess mucus that extends for an interval of 3 or more months each year for at least 2 consecutive years.

Emphysema: A severe lung disorder characterized by the gradual destruction of the tiny air sacs in the lung (alveoli) and a reduction in elasticity of lung tissue that impairs the lung's efficiency; the major symptom is a marked shortness of breath.

The walls of the air sacs are composed of blood-rich membranes that absorb the oxygen in the blood and dispense carbon dioxide into the air sacs for exhalation.

CHRONIC BRONCHITIS AND EMPHYSEMA

Chronic bronchitis and **emphysema** look very different from each other when viewed under a microscope. However, health-care professionals often refer to them together as *chronic obstructive pulmonary disease*, or COPD, and deemphasize their differences because each is rarely found in a pure form. They are also linked because they often occur at the same time and because both cause obstruction of the airways. A person with COPD usually has a combination of both chronic bronchitis and emphysema.

The major characteristic of chronic bronchitis is excessive mucus production. Typically, sufferers of the condition experience a cough and produce phlegm for at least 3 months of the year for 2 consecutive years. Doctors will make a diagnosis based on this history.

Emphysema is a degenerative lung disease characterized by a reduction in the number of air sacs and lessened elasticity of the remaining tissue. Upon exhalation, the lung tissue is more likely to collapse on itself, preventing the air from being exhaled. Technically, the diagnosis of emphysema can be made only from a biopsy. There are, however, some significant clues that signify its presence. Sufferers often lose a substantial amount of weight, for example, and their diminished breathing capacity is often evident during a physical examination. The lungs may also be hyperinflated, a condition a chest X ray can detect.

Causes of Chronic Bronchitis and Emphysema

Chronic bronchitis and emphysema usually result from a combination of genetic and environmental factors. Smoking, for example, is a major environmental factor and has been addressed previously. Other irritants known to cause lung problems include coal, asbestos, moldy hay, and chemicals. Why some people are more likely than others to develop chronic bronchitis or emphysema through contact with environmental elements is thought to be a result of genetics. For example, cigarette smoking substantially aggravates an inherited form of emphysema that is caused by an **antitrypsin enzyme deficiency**.

Symptoms and Diagnosis

Common symptoms of emphysema and chronic bronchitis include a chronic cough, sputum production, wheezing, and shortness of breath. Anyone suffering 1 of these 4 symptoms should see a doctor.

Doctors usually base a diagnosis of COPD upon a combination of personal history, reported symptoms, and a thorough physical examination. A chest X ray can help, not only by providing evidence of characteristic features of these illnesses but by excluding the possibility of pneumonia or lung cancer. Pulmo-

(continued on p. 91)

Antitrypsin enzyme deficiency: A deficiency in the lungs of a chemical known as alpha-antitrypsin that is thought to protect the lung tissue against emphysema; this deficiency appears to be genetic in origin.

It's Only a Cough

I sat in an armchair by my front window, making the most ghastly gasping sounds. It was the only way I could get any air into my lungs.

The ambulance arrived. An oxygen mask was clamped on my face, and I was sped to the emergency room—sirens wailing. The resident had me inhale from a bronchodilator, which contains drugs that relax the airways. Then, before sending me off for X rays and tests, she advised me to see a pulmonary specialist as soon as possible.

I did. And when I informed him I'd had a cough for over a year, he exclaimed, "You waited *this* long to come to a doctor?"

"I saw one," I said. "He told me lots of people have unexplained coughs. So I thought it was nothing to worry about."

The specialist shook his head. "Too many patients—*and* physicians—ignore the chronic cough. So often I've heard, 'It's only a cough. I've had it for years.' " He leaned forward. "Anyone who has a persistent cough for over three weeks *must* take it seriously."

He diagnosed my condition as asthmatic bronchitis, adding, "It's an obstructive pulmonary disease. Still, fortunately, reversible." He prescribed medication, bronchodilator therapy, and steroid spray four times a day to reduce inflammation of the airways. I left his office with the realization that if I hadn't had the emergency-room experience, I might well have lived with the cough until the term "reversible" was prefaced by those two ominous letters *ir.*

Startling Conclusions. My visit to the hospital prompted me to find out more about coughs. I discovered that they can be either "good" or "bad." The good cough gets rid of phlegm that encases bacteria. The bad, chronic cough can inflame the airways to such an extent that cough begets cough. The air passages become swollen and plugged, and infection may ensue.

[In May 1986,] I attended the annual meeting of the American Lung Association and its medical arm, the American Thoracic Society. After interviewing dozens of specialists, I came away with four startling conclusions about coughs:

1. A persistent cough is a clear warning that something is wrong. The most common ailment with persistent cough as a prime symptom is chronic bronchitis. This disease and its sister, emphysema, generally overlap. If you have one, you're likely to have the other to some degree. They've been classified together under the umbrella title Chronic Obstructive Pulmonary Disease, or COPD. Though the term is largely unknown to the public, COPD is the fastest-rising and fifth-leading cause of death in the country today. Ten million Americans suffer from it.

2. You can lose over 50 percent of your lungs to disease before symptoms show up. The lung is the largest organ in the body, containing six times the amount of tissue needed for normal breathing. The "unfolded" lungs of an average-sized adult would cover an entire tennis court.

This safety margin compensates for gradual loss of lung function through aging, but it also means that, according to Dr. Gareth Green, former president of the American Thoracic Society, "by the time you get symptoms, most of the damage may have been done." The key to treating lung disease is prevention, and that is why you *must* heed the warning signal of the chronic cough.

3. Doctors rarely use a readily available, inexpensive test that could warn patients in time for pulmonary diseases to be reversed or cured. A simple device called a spirometer, invented over 100 years ago, measures how well a person can expel air from the lungs. If used early, it can detect gradual lung deterioration due to COPD long before obvious symptoms that signal serious disability—such as chronic cough, excess sputum, unusual shortness of breath, and fatigue—appear. Dr. Reuben Cherniack, editor of *American Review of Respiratory Disease,* states: "The test should be given to every patient as part of a routine checkup. But few doctors perform the test, even though it takes less than a minute and requires minimal calculation."

4. Researchers and physicians have largely ignored the chronic cough. In 1970, when Dr. Richard Irwin was training in pulmonary disease at New York City's Columbia Presbyterian Hospital (he is now director of pulmonary medicine at the University of Massachusetts Medical School), a number of his patients had chronic coughs. But when he turned to the medical literature on the subject, he was "appalled" to find no step-by-step system to determine the cause of a chronic cough or the appropriate treatment.

Dr. Irwin then became one of the few pulmonary specialists to devote himself to the study of the chronic cough. His first contribution came about in 1977 because of a woman whose chronic cough had been diagnosed as psychogenic (all in the mind). A cough alone, with no wheezing or shortness of breath, could not be asthma, or so it said in the literature. Though the woman had no other symptoms, Irwin gave her an asthma test and she came out positive. He treated her with bronchodilator therapy used for asthmatics and, within a few days, the hacking cough she'd had for years completely disappeared. In 1979, after further research, Irwin and his colleagues published a paper alerting physicians to the fact that unexplained chronic cough could have a new diagnosis, easily pinpointed and contained: cough-equivalent asthma.

Irwin went on to investigate other chronic-cough causes, and in 1981 published a landmark paper describing specific methods of determining the most common causes of the persistent cough. "Once the diagnosis is accurately made," says Irwin, "there is an appropriate treatment for almost every cough-producing ailment—with rare exceptions such as late lung cancer. Unfortunately, by the time a cough is diagnosed as a symptom of lung cancer, it is almost always too late, even for surgery."

Causes of Chronic Coughs. Here are the most common reasons why people develop persistent coughs:

Chronic bronchitis. Many patients confuse chronic bronchitis, the prime disease having a chronic-cough component, with acute bronchitis, which can accompany a bad chest cold. Bronchitis becomes chronic when continual coughing results in such irritation that the inflamed airways become thickened and narrow. As the disease progresses, excessive mucus collects in the smaller airways or bronchioles, the "twigs" that branch off from the bronchial tubes like an upside-down tree. This obstruction can lead to the gasping-for-breath syndrome that landed me in the emergency room.

The main cause of chronic bronchitis is smoking, and environmental pollutants, allergies and certain viruses may aggravate it. With early diagnosis and proper medication, chronic bronchitis can be contained and some of its conditions reversed—*if* smoking is stopped.

Emphysema. Deep within the pulmonary tree—in the 600 million tiny air sacs called alveoli—"stale" carbon dioxide and "fresh" oxygen are exchanged. This crucial "gas exchange" is powered by elastin in the walls of the alveoli, which push the old air out. When emphysema sets in, lung tissue becomes like a worn-out girdle with no "push" left. The small airways narrow or collapse. Abnormally enlarged and filled with stagnant air, the alveoli give sufferers the desperate feeling of drowning. Symptoms can include chronic violent coughing. But emphysema's most crucial symptom is breathlessness.

Emphysema has long been classified "progressive and irreversible." However, new findings may change the gloomy picture. "There is now scientific evidence," says Dr. Thomas L. Petty, director of the Webb-Waring Lung Institute in Denver, "that if caught early enough, some of the components of the disease can be relieved."

The key word is *early.* "By the time a patient with emphysema or chronic bronchitis reports symptoms of altered lung function to a physician," Dr. Cherniack notes, "it's generally too late to prevent progression. Fifty to seventy percent die within five years."

The chief cause of emphysema? Smoking. In fact, smokers are six times as likely to die of emphysema as are non-smokers.

Asthma. Some eight million Americans suffer from asthma, which cannot be cured but *is* re-

versible with medication. Between attacks, patients can have normal or near-normal lung
function. Yet some 4000 people a year die from
asthma, and the death rate has been slowly
rising since 1979. A 1986 study showed that
fatalities among children and teen-agers have
doubled in the past decade.

Specialists often define asthma as "twitchy
airways"—the respiratory tubes overreact to al-
lergens or other irritants that don't trouble non-
asthmatics. In an attack, muscles around the
breathing tubes constrict, cells produce excess
mucus, and tissues lining the air passages swell,
making the opening for air pinpoint thin.

According to the American Lung Association,
asthma attacks can be as varied as fingerprints,
lasting anywhere from a few minutes to a few
weeks. Asthma may lie dormant for years—only
to emerge with a vengeance in later life.

"New" Diseases. There are a host of far less
prevalent but newly recognized cough-related
diseases. They have presumably existed for centuries, says Dr. James Gadek, director, pulmonary and critical-care division of Ohio State
University's College of Medicine. "What's new
and exciting is that researchers and clinicians
are finally identifying these diseases, developing
new ways to treat all of them and cure many of
them."

Bronchiolitis. This is an inflammation of the
hair-thin airways that connect the bronchi, or
large air tubes, to the microscopic air sacs. Until
recently it was thought to be an acute disease,
confined to children. Indeed, half of all hospitalized patients under two years old have bronchiolitis. "However," says Dr. Gadek, "we now
know that bronchiolitis can be a chronic adult
disease. It frequently comes on after a viral
illness and, if not properly diagnosed, can lead to
respiratory failure. But it is treatable with oral
steroids if their undesirable side effects can be
tolerated."

Allergic bronchopulmonary aspergillosis (ABPA).
Another recently recognized lung disease with a
chronic cough as its prime symptom may well
have existed since men lived in damp caves. Its

genesis is a fungus, aspergillus fumigatus,
whose spores are found in high concentrations in
musty basements, crawl spaces, compost heaps,
and marijuana. The fungus flourishes in warm,
dark climes—exactly the conditions provided by
the lungs. Studies suggest that people with
asthma or cystic fibrosis are especially vulnerable.

"If left untreated," says Dr. Paul Greenberger
of Northwestern University Medical School, "the
lungs will deteriorate—with no apparent symptoms other than a chronic cough."

The first test for the disease is a simple aller-
gist's "prick" test. People with ABPA develop an
immediate round, red reaction, known in allergy
parlance as "the wheal and flare." If subsequent
tests confirm ABPA, cortisone pills are prescribed. Within a year most patients are free of
fungal disease.

Ounce of Prevention. As part of your next
annual physical exam, ask your physician for a
baseline spirometer reading. Without regular
measurements, he will not be able to detect
gradual lung deterioration.

If you're a smoker, stop—whether or not you
have a cough. Dr. Robert Louden, a longtime
researcher of the chronic cough, points out,
"Cigarette smoking either causes or contributes
to many of the most important lung diseases."
But if you stop in time, your risk of developing
serious disease is greatly diminished.

Don't self-medicate a chronic cough. Far too
many do. Seek medical advice. "A chronic cough
is not a natural thing," says Dr. Gordon L. Snider,
president of the American Thoracic Society.
"Your lungs are trying to tell you something."

FOR INFORMATION on particular lung problems,
call the toll-free "hot line" of the National Jewish
Center for Immunology and Respiratory Medicine in Denver: 800-222-LUNG.

Source: Peggy Mann, Reader's Digest (November 1986),
pp. 21–28.

FIGURE 4.2
Portable Oxygen System

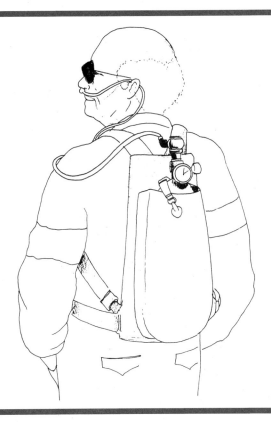

Portable oxygen units allow people with severe lung disease to continue with at least some of their regular activities. These units come in a wide range of sizes and styles, some weighing as little as five pounds.

nary function testing may also be necessary. **Pulmonary function tests** are a quantitative measure of the amount of air one can exhale over a given period. A blood test that measures the oxygen and carbon dioxide content of the blood may also be recommended. The blood test determines how well the lungs are functioning.

Treatment
First and foremost, those who smoke should quit immediately once chronic bronchitis or emphysema has been diagnosed. The

Pulmonary function tests: Breathing tests that measure several aspects of the respiratory cycle, including the amount of air exhaled and the force of expiration to help determine if there is any impediment to the flow of air to or from the lungs.

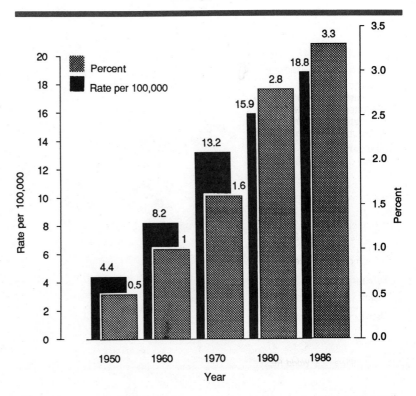

FIGURE 4.3
COPD Mortality from 1950–1986

Legend:
- Percent
- Rate per 100,000

Source: *Journal of the American Medical Association*, Vol. 264, No. 24, 26 December 1990, p. 3181.

Bronchodilators: A group of drugs that widen the airways in the lungs and are used to treat a variety of conditions in which the flow of air into the lungs is obstructed or reduced.

Anticholinergic drugs: A group of drugs that block the action of acetylcholine, a neurotransmitter that stimulates cell activity, thus relieving a range of symptoms, including the excessive contraction of the bronchioles associated with asthma.

Theophylline: A bronchodilator that is primarily used in the treatment of asthma.

Lung disease, excluding lung cancer, is the fifth most common cause of death in the United States. This chart shows how Chronic Obstructive Pulmonary Disease (COPD) deaths have increased since 1950.

treatment for these diseases will not cure them but will relieve their symptoms. Medication may be necessary to decrease the production of phlegm. Today doctors will use **bronchodilators**, **anticholinergic drugs**, and **theophylline** agents to treat COPD sufferers. These are now more commonly prescribed than therapies that merely reduce phlegm. In addition, treating COPD means preventing other conditions that can cause complications. For example, flu and pneumonia are much more serious illnesses

FIGURE 4.4
Asthma Treatment

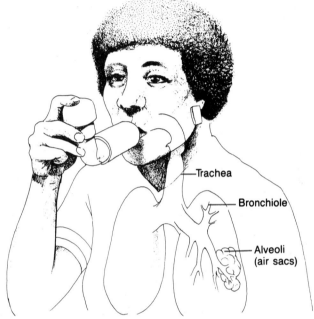

Bronchodilators

These drugs reopen airways.

Beta$_2$-agonists
- Albuterol *(Proventil, Ventolin, Volmax)*
- Bitolterol mesylate *(Tomalate)*
- Pirbuterol *(Maxair)*
- Terbutaline *(Brethine, Brethaire, Bricanyl)*

Methylxanthines
- Theophylline *(Marax, Quibron, Theo-Dur)*

Anti-inflammatory drugs

They prevent swelling inside airways.

Steroids
- Beclomethasone *(Beclovent, Vanceril)*
- Flunisolide *(AeroBid)*
- Prednisone
- Triamcinolone acetonide *(Azmecort)*

Anti-allergy drugs
- Cromolyn sodium *(Intal)*

Names in italics are brand names.

Trachea

Bronchiole

Alveoli
(air sacs)

Source: *U.S. News & World Report*, 4 March 1991, p. 61.

The drugs most often prescribed for treating asthma are bronchodilators, which reopen the bronchioles, and anti-inflammatory drugs, which prevent swelling inside the airways. These drugs can either be inhaled, as shown in this illustration, or taken orally.

among those with underlying lung disease. Flu shots and pneumonia shots become very important. Supplemental oxygen and medication may be called for to help maximize the lungs' ability to function.

If it reaches its final stage, lung disease may require the continuous use of oxygen. This includes home-oxygen delivery systems and portable systems to allow people to continue with usual activities as much as possible. Even then, life may be far from normal. For example, marked sensitivity to smoke may exclude lung disease victims from many public places. They may also move slowly, have coughing fits, and endure the embarrassment associated with tending to their special needs.

OCCUPATIONAL LUNG DISEASES

Experts suggest that at least 100,000 Americans are at risk of contracting lung diseases associated with occupational exposure to risk factors. [3] The extent of these diseases is difficult to pinpoint because the onset of an occupational disease can occur many years after initial exposure to risk factors. That makes it difficult for doctors to distinguish between illnesses that begin in the workplace and those that develop from other causes. Nevertheless, the benefit in understanding these diseases is clear: Decreased exposure is likely to lead to fewer and less severe cases of lung disease associated with the workplace.

What Are the Occupational Lung Diseases?

Occupational lung disease is a label applied to a group of lung and respiratory problems caused by the inhalation of particles or chemicals while at work. When this happens, the lung has only a few ways in which to respond. The lung tissue may scar, a condition known as **fibrosis**, so that oxygen can't cross the membranes into the blood. Bronchitis or asthma-like symptoms may appear. Illness resembling pneumonia may occur. Cancer can develop. Exposure to certain organic proteins may cause an allergic form of pneumonia.

Although their causes are different, many of these diseases have similar symptoms. Because some occur with frequency and regularity, they have been named after the known cause. [4] For example, coal miner's lung, or black lung, results from inhaling coal dust in the mining process. Symptoms of this disease are similar to those of chronic bronchitis and can be more severe if the sufferer smokes.

Asbestos, a common form of inorganic dust, is actually a general term for several different kinds of silicate minerals. Experts have identified asbestos exposure as a cause of occupational lung disease. More than 9.1 million Americans who have been exposed to asbestos in the workplace are alive today and are at risk of developing lung disease. Because asbestos has been so widely used in construction and in many other industries, it has affected many people in a wide range of occupations. Experts believe that those at risk include not only the workers but their families, who may have been exposed to asbestos dust that has clung to the workers' clothing. Other groups of workers at risk for occupational lung disease include those in the quartz mining, china clay processing, and metal grinding and casting industries.

Fibrosis: Any overgrowth of scar or connective tissue, particularly one which replaces normal surrounding tissue; such overgrowths can significantly impair vital body functions when they occur in specialized organs such as the lungs.

ASTHMA

Asthma, an intermittent, reversible, reactive respiratory disease, causes gasping and wheezing and a feeling of constriction in the chest. This response is called an episode or "asthma attack" and is really an allergic reaction. Asthmatics inherit a hyperresponsive bronchial tree, also known as "twitchy lungs." Different things will provoke an asthma response in different people.

(continued on p. 98)

Asthma: An abrupt or chronic condition characterized by narrowed airways within the lungs, which causes obstruction of the airflow.

Asthma Triggers: Know Your Troublemakers

WHAT CAUSES ASTHMA?

Asthma is caused by extra sensitive lungs that over-react to certain factors. Those factors, or asthma "triggers," vary widely among asthma sufferers.

An important step in getting control of your asthma is to discover those factors or combinations of factors that trigger asthma episodes in your lungs.

The more you know about your own personal asthma troublemakers, the better you will be able to work with your doctor to prevent and control asthma episodes.

What do you think your asthma triggers are? Write them [down], then see if you think of others as you read on.

TRIGGER: ALLERGIES

Is asthma caused by allergies?

There is allergic and non-allergic asthma. When the cause of asthma is allergies, they usually, though not always, appear before age 35.

If you have allergic asthma, your lungs will go into an asthma state when you contact things you are allergic to.

If I never had allergies as a child, could I get them now?

Yes. Allergies can take many years to develop. A change in your lifestyle such as a new job or a move to a new area could have exposed you to new causes. And asthma patterns can change with age.

What could I be allergic to?

The list is almost endless. Some common culprits are the tiny particles, including pollens and mold spores, that get into the air from trees, plants, and hay.

Animal skin, hair, and feathers, including wool clothing and feather pillows, also give off tiny particles that can cause allergies.

Insect parts such as particles from dead cockroaches are a major problem, especially in cities.

Asthma can be caused by allergies to foods such as nuts, chocolate, eggs, orange juice, fish, or milk.

Some people are sensitive to certain substances without being allergic. For example, asthma in some people is triggered by sulfites; this preservative may be sprayed on or added to fresh fruits and vegetables, shellfish, beer, and wine. Another chemical trigger for some people with asthma is aspirin.

If I have allergic asthma, what can I do?

The first thing is for you and your doctor to find out what things trigger your allergic asthma.

Then, because each patient is different, the doctor may try different treatments to see what works best. He or she may ask you to try to avoid the things you are allergic to . . . or give you injections to help make you less sensitive to those things . . . or treat you with medicines that help prevent asthma episodes despite your allergies.

TRIGGER: HOUSEHOLD PRODUCTS

When I work at home, I sometimes have asthma trouble. What household products can trigger asthma?

Our homes are loaded with products that can irritate the sensitive lungs of asthma sufferers and bring on episodes. Try to avoid breathing vapors from cleaning solvents, paint, paint thinner, and liquid chlorine bleach.

Also avoid household sprays such as furniture polish, starch, and cleaners.

Personal products in the home also can irritate your lungs. Common troublemakers are spray deodorants, perfumes, hair sprays, talcum powder, and scented cosmetics.

Reactions to these products may be mild or severe. Some people are helped by using baking soda in water or special baking soda cleaning products for household cleaning. Some jobs, like painting, may have to be done by someone else.

Even if you notice little or no reaction from household products, it's best for everyone with asthma to avoid sprays and breathe the cleanest air possible.

TRIGGER: DUSTS

Do I need to avoid household dust?

Many people with mild or medically controlled asthma need to take no special care to avoid ordinary dust. However, some people are very sensitive to dust of any kind. And certain kinds of dusts can be asthma triggers.

If you have severe reactions to household dust, try to avoid breathing it by:

- Avoiding household furnishings that raise dust when they are used, like draw drapes and cloth-upholstered furniture.
- Dusting your surroundings frequently, before much dust accumulates. Use a damp cloth.
- Damp-mopping floors instead of sweeping.

Too much dust may be raised by using a vacuum cleaner. Some people need to leave the room while this job is being done.

Clean filters on hot air furnaces and on air conditioners help keep dust out of the air.

Some people are helped by making a special effort to keep a dust-free bedroom. The room can be furnished without carpet, draperies, knick-knacks, or other dust collectors.

TRIGGER: ON THE JOB

What other kinds of dusts or fumes can trigger asthma?

Some people who may have no trouble with house dust can develop asthma from breathing certain dusts, gases, or vapors at work. This can happen immediately or it may take years.

Work products that have been known to cause asthma in some workers include:

- Wood products such as western red cedar, some pine and birch woods, and mahogany. These are used by woodworkers and some farm workers.
- Organic dusts such as flour, cereals, grains, coffee and tea dust, and papain dust from meat tenderizer. These can affect millers, bakers, and food processors.
- Metals such as platinum, chromium, nickel sulfate, and soldering fumes. Workers in refining and manufacturing operations may have trouble with these.
- Gases and aerosols including sulfur dioxide breathed by brewery workers, fumigators, refrigeration workers, and others; chlorine gas by petrochemical workers in refineries; nitrogen dioxide by diesel operators; and fluorocarbon propellants by beauticians.
- Cotton, flax, and hemp dust inhaled by workers in cotton processing and textile industries. This asthma-like condition also is known as byssinosis or brown lung disease.
- Mold from decaying hay can trigger asthma in farmers.

What can I do about air pollution?

- Avoid places with very dirty air, such as traffic jams, parking garages, dusty work areas, and smoke-filled rooms.

- Avoid breathing in smoke from cigarettes, pipes, and cigars. Ask smokers to respect your need for clean air.
- During times of heavy smog, check your radio or television news for air pollution alerts.

What should I do on days when air pollution is heavy?

With good medical care, most asthma sufferers are able to carry on a normal schedule in spite of air pollution. But days when the air is hot, humid, and dirty can slow down anyone.

If heavy pollution tends to trigger asthma episodes in you, discuss this problem in advance with your doctor. Plan to prevent an episode from happening. Your doctor may recommend extra medicine for those times, or a change in activities.

You will breathe in less pollution if you stay indoors with the windows closed, and circulate air with a fan or air conditioner. Relax and avoid heavy work and dust-raising activities until the excess pollution lifts.

Always avoid strenuous outdoor exercise during periods of heavy air pollution.

TRIGGER: EXERCISE

I have trouble with asthma after I've been working hard or playing sports. Can exercise be an asthma trigger?

It is for some people. Some asthma sufferers begin wheezing after they overexert themselves—running upstairs too fast, carrying heavy loads, jogging, bikeriding, or playing team sports, for example.

Do I have to give up some activities?

Your goal should be to live a normal life. Exercise is important for your general health and for your lungs. If the form of exercise you enjoy triggers asthma, ask your doctor about taking medicine in advance to prevent episodes.

You may need to adjust your pace a bit, taking the stairs a little slower, or trying out a different sport. Swimming works especially well for many asthma sufferers.

TRIGGER: INFECTIONS

Do colds and infections cause asthma episodes?

Colds and infections can make asthma worse. Virus infections, especially, are known asthma triggers. You can't avoid coming in contact with germs that may cause infection, but you can help your body fight them off if you follow these steps:

- Ask your doctor if you need flu and pneumonia vaccinations.
- Keep your body healthy with daily exercise, nourishing foods, and enough sleep so that you're better able to fight off the germs that cause infections.
- Keep your lungs as clear of mucus as you can. Drink enough fluids.

What are the danger signs of infection?

Suspect an infection, and call your doctor if you notice one of these:

- You have fever or chills.
- You're more short of breath, or you're wheezing more than usual.
- Your cough is worse than usual.
- You have more mucus, or it's thicker than usual, or the color changes.
- You lose your appetite, feel dizzy or sleepy, or have headaches.

What should I do if I have an infection?

- Take the medicine your doctor orders exactly as directed. Don't stop before your doctor says to, even if you feel better.
- Carefully follow your doctor's directions for clearing your lungs of mucus.
- Report right away to your doctor if your condition gets worse.
- Keep small infections from growing large. Give your doctor time to treat them before they spread.

TRIGGER: NIGHTTIME

My asthma episodes almost always happen at night. Does sleeping cause asthma?

Nighttime asthma is common. While you sleep your airways may become narrow and collect mucus. This kind of asthma responds to normal treatment and may be prevented by taking medicine before bedtime.

Another nighttime problem for many asthma sufferers is bringing up stomach contents into the throat. This can be helped by raising the head of the bed, eating small meals, and avoiding lying down for two hours after eating. Taking antacids at night may also help.

Your doctor can advise you on ways to manage your nighttime asthma problems.

TRIGGER: EMOTIONS

Can asthma be caused by emotions?

At one time it was commonly believed that asthma was the body's way of expressing an emotional problem. But now we can say for sure that asthma is not caused by emotions or by mental problems. However, emotions can play a role, as they can in almost any illness.

How can my emotions affect my asthma?

Strong emotions can affect anyone's breathing. You've heard people say, "I was so *scared* I couldn't breathe," or, "She was breathless with *excitement*," or perhaps you've used the term "breathing easier" to express the feeling of *relief.*

For some people with asthma, strong emotions can cause trouble in several ways. For example:

- Expressing emotions by laughing, crying, or yelling can stimulate nerves that cause muscles in your airways to tighten.
- Fear during an asthma episode may cause you to breathe too hard and fast—and that can make the episode worse.
- Sometimes people with asthma become angry and frustrated, and refuse to take the medicines that can prevent episodes.

Source: *The Asthma Handbook* (New York: American Lung Association, 1984), pp. 4–8.

Some asthmatics are allergic to hay, grasses, or animal dander. In others, smoke or air pollution trigger the same response. In still others, an upper respiratory infection may set off the attack. Asthma attacks may also occur without a specific stimulus. Regardless of the stimulus, during an attack respiratory muscles narrow, tissue becomes inflamed, and phlegm gathers in the bronchioles. Asthma frequently begins early in life (many people suffer their first attack before the age of 5), but it can develop at any age. It appears to be equally prevalent among all races and both genders. [5]

Symptoms and Diagnosis

An asthma diagnosis can be based on the presence of certain characteristic symptoms. These include an intermittent cough, wheezing, and shortness of breath. These symptoms typically happen suddenly, occur at night, may be mild or severe, and gradually improve with time. Between episodes, the asthma sufferer may exhibit no symptoms. During these periods, a pul-

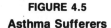

FIGURE 4.5
Asthma Sufferers

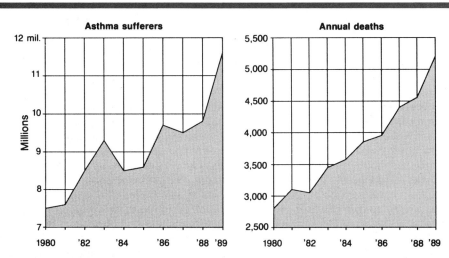

Source: *U.S. News and World Report,* 4 March 1991, p. 61.

About 1 in 21 Americans, or some 11.6 million people, have asthma. From 1980 to 1989 the percentage of asthma sufferers has increased 55 percent, and the percentage of deaths from asthma has increased an average of 6 percent.

monary function test can help a doctor make an asthma diagnosis.

Treatment

If the asthma is triggered by a known allergen, removing or avoiding that allergen is the best treatment. If an episode is triggered by infection, antibiotics may be necessary. Medications that help to reduce inflammation, called **corticosteroids**, may be inhaled or given orally. Doctors can also prescribe medications that dilate the bronchioles. It is also worth noting that most children who suffer asthma outgrow their symptoms by the age of 21 and live their adult lives asthma free.

INFECTIONS: COLDS, FLU, AND PNEUMONIA

The term "cold" actually refers to a group of illnesses caused by viruses that invade the upper respiratory tract. These viruses are

(continued on p. 103)

Did You Know That . . .

More than 10 million Americans have asthma, of which three million are children. The disease tends to run in families, and most sufferers also have allergies.

Corticosteroids: Hormonal preparations that help to diminish inflammation; they are used to treat a variety of conditions, including asthma.

A Practical Approach to the Emotions and Asthma

Some years ago, I had the grandiose hope that perhaps I could help discover a psychological cure for the disease called asthma. At that time, asthma was still widely thought to be psychosomatic. Scientists and the public alike thought that asthma was not truly a physical problem in the same sense as is, say, viral pneumonia but rather the patient's way of expressing in body language his underlying emotional problem.

Some people believed that asthma existed primarily in the patient's mind or that the patient could voluntarily control it. Others had the idea that asthma was a bad habit—something like temper tantrums, a habit learned in order to get attention from an indifferent or rejecting environment. In general, it was taken for granted, as it had been for over a thousand years, that the key to asthma would be found hidden in the complexities of the patient's personality.

In the past decade, scientific studies have discredited these ideas. We know now that asthma is a bona fide medical illness, the basic nature and origin of which, while not fully understood, are undoubtedly physical. We know also that psychological factors *are* important components of the disease but in the sense that they are able to increase or decrease the frequency and severity of episodes.

Emotions and behavior

There are four different ways in which emotions and behavior can influence the course of asthma.

The first is the simplest and also the rarest. It is the instance in which an asthma episode is directly triggered by emotions. A good example was reported to me by a young patient of mine. I'll call her Mary. Mary was 11 years old when she told me that, when she learned that she had been elected president of her Girl Scout troop, she felt a surge of excitement run through her body and almost immediately felt her chest begin to tighten up. She then went through an asthma episode.

Another example is reflected in the experience of a teenage girl who told me that one of her most horrifying experiences is to discover that she has forgotten her medication when she's away from home. The more she worries about it, she says, the worse her asthma gets. This kind of emotionally induced asthma is, in my experience, relatively rare. Much more common are the following patterns.

In the second pattern, the patient experiences an emotion which is followed at some point by an episode of asthma. However, unlike the first instance, it isn't the emotion per se that precipitates the asthma but what the person does about it. For example, an asthmatic child gets angry and storms and stomps about. The overexertion involved, rather than the anger itself, can trigger an asthma episode. Or, if a patient is afraid that his friends will find out that he has asthma and avoids taking medication, he may suffer unnecessarily frequent or severe episodes of asthma. The asthma episodes occur not because he is self-conscious about his disease but because of what he does in response to his self-consciousness.

In the third pattern, behavior or emotions induce asthma, but it is neither the emotion nor the behavior per se that sets off the episode. Rather, it is those things with which the behavior brings the patient in contact that provokes symptoms. A simple example is the child, allergic to animal dander, who angrily refuses to follow medical advice and plays with dogs and cats. It is not the anger that brings on the asthma, nor is it the playing that does it. Instead, the allergen with which the child comes in contact results in the onset of symptoms.

Finally, there is the fourth pattern in which the patient gets asthma for whatever reason. Then, the way the patient or the people around him react to the asthma affects the course of the episode. A common example is the patient who is frightened by his asthma.

Which of these patterns is operating will, of

course, vary from patient to patient and across time for any one patient.

The patterns can be reversed

So far, I have described four negative patterns in which emotions or behavior trigger or aggravate asthma. However, for each negative pattern there is a positive counterpart. For example, in the first case, where emotions such as excitement or fear trigger asthma episodes, relaxation can help the patient to avoid or to minimize asthma episodes. Relaxation has even been shown to have a temporary bronchodilating effect.

Similarly, in the second pattern, patients can be taught ways of expressing feelings that do not trigger an asthma episode. In the third example, the patient can be helped to come into contact with things that please him but do not set off an episode. And in the fourth illustration, the patient and his family can be taught to react to asthma symptoms adaptably and calmly.

Thus, by identifying the patterns at work in a given patient and helping him and his family to substitute a positive counterpart, we help the patient to discover that a certain amount of his symptoms can be avoided. In effect, we teach the patient to think and to act in terms of preventive self-help.

So it is possible to help patients to avoid a certain amount of their symptoms in reasonably clear-cut ways. Unfortunately, it often takes a surprising amount of work to make people want to use them. Some patients and their families feel so anxious or helpless about the illness that they would rather depend upon a professional for help. Very often, the anxiety and helplessness result from inadequate knowledge or understanding about asthma and its causes. Sometimes other pressures prevent people from helping themselves. Teenagers, for example, often hide or deny their asthma and avoid learning self-help techniques because they are afraid of being found out and rejected.

Anxiety and helplessness are not genetic components of asthma. Being unable to breathe freely certainly can be a frightening sensation, but the amount of anxiety can be minimized or enhanced by the family's reactions. Parents who are frightened and parents who are calm when the child gets asthma will inculcate in the child very different reactions to symptoms. Parents who feel guilty or ashamed or who behave in haphazard ways are going to inculcate shame and haphazardness in their children. In like manner, parents who model self-control, consistency, and a straightforward approach to dealing with asthma symptoms will make it easier for their child to react similarly.

Family asthma programs can help

Parents are not the only important role models for children. During the past few years, family asthma programs, many of them organized and sponsored by lung associations, have sprung up in various parts of the country. These programs are designed to provide an important group experience and an important psychological experience as well. The children are exposed to other children who have already learned that asthma need not induce fear. Such children—or asthmatic adults who are sports or business figures—should be very deliberately included in the group. They can help demonstrate to the frightened or apathetic or oppositional child that asthma need not be more than merely a part of his life and that it is a part over which he can have a good deal of control.

With encouragement and exposure to positive role models, the asthmatic child can learn to gauge and to handle physical stress appropriately. Typically, the problem asthmatic mishandles physical stress in one of two ways. Either he avoids physical exertion because he's afraid of getting sick, or, for whatever reason, he overdoes the exertion and winds up getting sick unnecessarily. In a group situation, such a child can learn appropriate physical limits while coming to appreciate his real capacities.

The group can also benefit the asthmatic child who is openly frightened by his illness or who conceals his anxieties behind a mask of denial. The opportunity to see other children with the same illness and to share experiences with them can be dramatically supportive. This effect has been documented not only in children but in adults as well. Sharing experiences with other asthmatics and learning how they handle their disease have been found to result in fewer visits to emergency rooms, fewer days missed at work or at school, and, in positive terms, a generally better sense of well-being.

What makes the group so potentially useful for teaching adaptive patterns is that informed and sympathetic people can be on hand to reward the child for efforts to change in the right direction. Families can help in this, and family asthma programs can help them do it well. Too frequently, we see families criticize the asthmatic child for doing what's wrong, but they fall short in reinforcing the child for attempts to handle his problems well.

The asthma group, then, can be a setting for the open exchange of accurate information on the disease, for reinforced practice of new ways of living with asthma, and for learning to relax with the disease while also learning how to avoid it as much as is reasonable. But these desirable components need to be deliberately and thoughtfully designed into the asthma programs if they are to be maximally effective.

Asthma—a problem for an athlete

I would like to close with a little success story. It is about a young man—we'll call him Jack—who was one of my patients. I first saw him when he was 15 years old. He'd had asthma since about the age of 6 and had had a two-year spontaneous remission when he was 9. Since age 11, his asthma had been chronic, with some seasonal variations. Episodes of his asthma were triggered by foods, dust, odors, worries about school, and fears of getting asthma. They were also triggered at times when he was alone in his room, wishing he could be out playing sports, and, ironically, they were triggered by overexertion when he did compete.

The year after Jack's asthma had come back, when he was 11, Jack told himself that there was no way he was going back to being an asthmatic who couldn't play and who was rejected by his friends. He decided he was going to play no matter what the cost and that he was going to hide his asthma. If his breathing became labored

in the middle of a football game, Jack would pretend his ankle was hurting so he could sit down and rest; he wouldn't admit he was having a hard time breathing. At other times, he'd medicate himself heavily at the least suspicion of an episode, or, if he thought he might get symptoms, he'd take extra medication in advance. (Such preventive use of medicine is not necessarily bad. In Jack's case, however, it was overdone.)

Jack turned out to be a gifted athlete, and by the time I saw him, he was a muscular five-foot-ten star in almost every competitive sport. But he was also having a lot of asthma. He had reached the point where sports were an obsession. They were rarely out of his mind, and, if he couldn't play, he worried. He confided that he secretly wished he could tell his friend, "I don't want to play today." So far, however, he hadn't dared.

A program for Jack

The treatment we did with Jack was straightforward. We designed a program with three goals: 1) help Jack to relax; 2) teach him to be assertive with his friends—to say, "Look, I don't want to play today"; and 3) teach Jack to find alternate sports, like bowling, that he could play on days when he didn't feel up to the strenuous ones.

In addition to teaching Jack these things, we also took measurements. Using a peak flow meter in his house, Jack measured the limits of his lung function three times a day. We called him each day to get the measurements as well as a report on how much medication he'd taken in the past 24 hours and how bad he thought his asthma had been. We also asked whether he had been exposed to any of the things that would precipitate an asthma episode.

The great variability in Jack's lung function before treatment showed up clearly on the peak flow record. He was having asthmatic symptoms almost daily. When his peak flow went down, Jack's medication intake and his subjective estimate of asthma would go up.

For three or four weeks, we did nothing but observe. Then we started to work with Jack toward the goals I described. We worked with him on relaxation techniques; we gave him assertiveness training; and we began to convince him that he could choose from a variety of sports, strenuous and nonstrenuous, depending upon how he felt.

What happened as Jack went through the program was documented by the peak flow record and by Jack's own reports. The sharp variations in his lung function began to level off. The amount of medication he took dropped off and stabilized. And the amount of suffering—Jack's subjective asthma severity—declined considerably. He worried less and overexerted himself less. He had learned self-help through self-control.

Key to self-help

The key to self-help is confidence in one's ability to exert control. In this connection, it would be hard to overestimate the impact that asthma programs can have on children who have learned to think of themselves as different, helpless, and inferior.

The degree to which such programs can contribute to enhanced self-confidence and pride is, to my way of thinking, a prime measure of their value. The self-esteem, the confidence, and the restored perspective that an asthma program can engender in children need to be seen to be appreciated. Those of you who have seen the results don't need any further convincing by me. To those of you who have not seen them, I urge you to go out and see for yourself.

Source: Jonathan H. Weiss, *American Lung Association Bulletin* (June 1982), pp. 1–4.

usually contracted during the colder months of the year, when people are indoors and in close proximity. The virus is present on the infected person's skin and also in droplets he or she may cough or sneeze into the air. Typically, the virus is spread through hand-to-hand contact, either directly, through touching an infected person, or indirectly, through handling infected objects, such as playing cards. The best way to prevent a cold is to keep your hands away from your face and wash your hands after touching someone known to have one. Young children and their parents typically get 6 to 12 colds per year. Older adults may get as few as 2 or 3 colds per year, or even none at all.

Influenza, or "the flu" as it is more commonly known, is also caused by a group of respiratory viruses that infect and inflame the tissues lining the respiratory tract. In healthy adults and children, the flu is typically a moderate illness that lasts only a week. But it is a far more serious illness for a person with underlying health problems. Such victims are more likely to have complications that could prove fatal even if properly treated. The complications are usually bacterial infections that occur when the body's immune-system defenses are weakened and can lead to serious diseases, such as **bacterial pneumonia**. In an epidemic year, 20 to 30 percent of the population may get the flu. People who have other chronic illnesses at the time of an outbreak

Influenza: A viral respiratory infection popularly known as the "flu"; the symptoms of influenza include fever, chills, headache, muscle ache, loss of appetite, and general weakness.

Bacterial pneumonia: An inflammation of the lungs caused by bacterial infection; the major symptoms of pneumonia include fever, chills, shortness of breath, and, in more severe cases, the coughing up of sputum or blood.

Did You Know That . . .

The name "influenza" came about in the Middle Ages when people believed the disease was influenced by the stars.

FIGURE 4.6
Invasion of the Influenza Virus

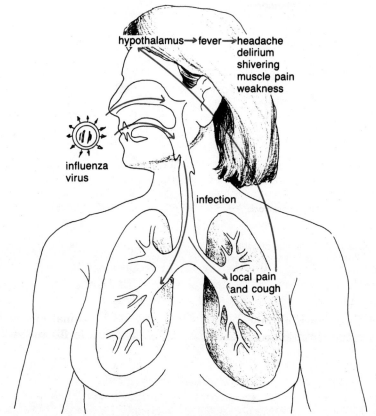

Source: Andrew Scott, *Pirates of the Cell* (Basil Blackwell, 1985), p. 112.

The influenza virus enters the body through the mouth or nasal cavity and can inflame and infect the tissues of the respiratory system. The most common symptoms are local pain and coughing, headache, fever, weakness, shivering, and delirium.

appear to be particularly susceptible and are more likely to have complications. It is recommended that those at increased risk have a yearly flu shot either to reduce the likelihood of getting the flu in the first place or to reduce its severity. People at risk include:

FIGURE 4.7
Lobar and Bronchial Pneumonia

Lobar pneumonia   **Bronchial pneumonia**

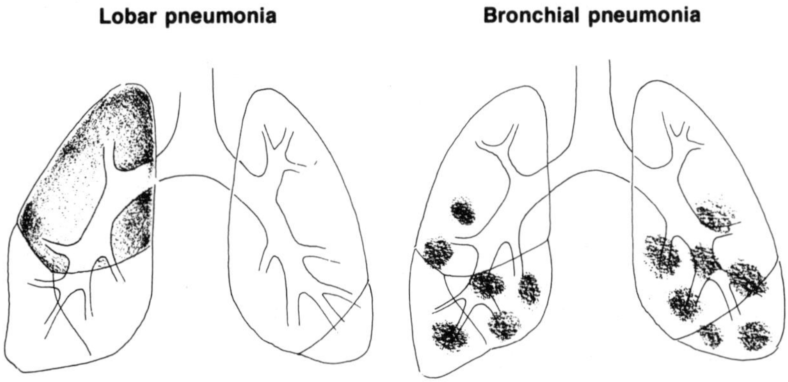

Source: *Facts About Pneumonia* (New York: American Lung Association, 1988), p. 2.

Pneumonia is the name of not one but a number of diseases with similar symptoms. The illustration above shows the difference between lobar and bronchial pneumonia.

1. Those with chronic lung disease, such as asthma, emphysema, chronic bronchitis, tuberculosis, or **cystic fibrosis**

2. Those with heart disease

3. Those who suffer chronic kidney disease

4. Those who have diabetes or other chronic metabolic disorders

5. Those with severe anemia

6. Those who have a disease or treatment regimen that depresses immunity

7. Residents in a nursing home or other chronic care facility

8. Those aged 65 and older

9. Physicians, nurses, or other providers of care to high-risk persons. [6]

Pneumonia is an illness characterized by inflammation of either one or both lungs, which then fill with fluid, pus, or mucus.

(continued on p. 108)

Cystic fibrosis: A genetically inherited disease characterized by excessive mucus production by the lining of the bronchial tubes and an inability to digest fats; although a variety of treatments are now available, cystic fibrosis remains a serious and ultimately life-threatening disease.

Facts About Pneumonia

What Is Pneumonia?

Pneumonia is a serious infection or inflammation of your lungs. The air sacs in the lungs fill with pus, and other liquid. Oxygen has trouble reaching your blood. If there is too little oxygen in your blood, your body cells can't work properly—and may die.

Pneumonia Is On The Rise

Until 1936, pneumonia was the No. 1 cause of death in the U.S. Then antibiotics brought it under control. Now this deadly enemy is making a comeback, in part because some bacteria can resist antibiotics. Pneumonia and influenza combined have ranked as the sixth leading cause of death since 1979.

Causes Of Pneumonia

Pneumonia is not a single disease. It can have over 30 different causes.

There are four main causes of pneumonia:

1. Bacteria

2. Viruses

3. Mycoplasmas

4. Others, such as pneumocystis

1. Bacterial Pneumonia

Bacterial pneumonia can attack anyone from infants through the very old. Alcoholics, the debilitated, post-operative patients, people with respiratory diseases or viral infections and people who are immunocompromised are particularly vulnerable.

The *pneumococcus* is the most common cause of bacterial pneumonia. It is the only form of pneumonia for which a vaccine is available.

How Bacterial Pneumonia Strikes

Pneumonia bacteria are present in some healthy throats. When body defenses are weakened in some way—by illness, old age, malnutrition, general debility, impaired immunity—the bacteria can multiply and do serious damage. Usually when a person's resistance is lowered, bacteria work their way into the lungs and inflame the air sacs. The tissue of part of a lobe of the lung, an entire lobe, or even most of the lungs' five lobes becomes completely filled with liquid matter. (This is called "consolidation.") The infection quickly spreads through the bloodstream and the whole body is invaded.

Symptoms: The onset of bacterial pneumonia can vary from gradual to sudden. The patient may experience shaking chills, chattering, severe chest pain, and a cough that produces rust-colored or greenish sputum. Temperature often shoots up as high as 105. The patient sweats profusely, and his [or her] breathing and pulse rate increase rapidly. From lack of oxygen in the blood, his [or her] lips and nailbeds may have a bluish cast. His [or her] mental state may be clouded or delirious.

2. Viral Pneumonia

Half of all pneumonias are believed to be of viral origin. More and more viruses are being identified as the cause of respiratory infection, and though most attack the upper respiratory tract, some produce pneumonia, especially in children. Most of these pneumonias are patchy and self-limiting, but *primary influenza virus* may be severe and occasionally fatal. The virus invades the lungs and multiplies, but there are almost no physical signs of lung tissue becoming filled with fluid. It finds most of its victims among those who have preexisting heart or pulmonary illness or are pregnant.

Symptoms: The initial symptoms of viral pneumonia are those of influenza: fever, a dry cough, headache, muscle pain, and weakness. Within 12 to 36 hours, there is increasing breathlessness, the cough becomes worse and produces a scant amount of bloody sputum. There is a high fever and there may be blueness of lips. In the final stage, the patient has unbearable air hunger and breathlessness. Other viral pneumonias are complicated by an invasion of bacteria—with all the typical symptoms of *bacterial* pneumonia.

3. Mycoplasma Pneumonia

Because of its symptoms and physical signs, and because the course of the illness differed strikingly from those of classic pneumococcal pneumonia, mycoplasma pneumonia was once believed to be caused by one or more undiscovered viruses and was called "primary atypical pneumonia."

Identified during World War II, mycoplasmas are the smallest free-living agents of disease in man, unclassified as to whether bacteria or viruses, but having characteristics of both. They generally cause a mild and widespread pneumonia. It affects all age groups, occurring most frequently in older children and young adults. The death rate is low, even in untreated cases.

Symptoms: The most prominent symptom of mycoplasma pneumonia is a cough that tends to come in violent paroxysms, but produces only sparse whitish sputum. Chilly sensations and fever are early symptoms, and some patients experience nausea or vomiting. The patient's heartbeat is often slow, and in some extreme cases he [or she] may suffer from breathlessness and have a bluish cast to his [or her] lips and nailbeds.

4. Other Kinds Of Pneumonia

Pneumocystis carinii pneumonia (PCP) is caused by an organism long thought of as a parasite but now believed to be a fungus. PCP is the first sign of illness in more than half of all persons with AIDS, and perhaps 80 percent (four out of five) will develop it sooner or later. It can be successfully treated in many cases. It may recur a few months later, but treatment can help to prevent or delay its recurrence.

Many of the less common pneumonias have a high death toll and are occurring more often. Various special pneumonias are caused by the inhalation of food, liquid, gases, dust, or a foreign body, by fungi, or by a bronchial obstruction such as a tumor. Rickettsia (also considered something between viruses and bacteria) cause Rocky Mountain spotted fever, Q fever, typhus, and psittacosis—diseases that involve the lungs to a greater or lesser extent. Tuberculosis pneumonia is an overwhelming lung infection and extremely dangerous unless treated early.

Treatment Of Pneumonia

If you develop pneumonia, your chances of prompt recovery are greatest under certain conditions: if you're young, if your pneumonia was caught early, if your defenses against disease are working well, if the infection hasn't spread, and if you're not suffering from other illness.

In the young and healthy, prompt treatment with antibiotics can cure bacterial and mycoplasma pneumonia, and a certain percentage of rickettsia cases. There is no effective treatment yet for viral pneumonia.

The drug or drugs used are determined by the germ causing the pneumonia and the judgement of the physician. After temperature returns to normal, medication must be continued according to physician's instructions—otherwise the pneumonia may recur. Relapses can be far more serious than the first attack.

Besides antibiotics, patients are given supportive treatment: proper diet, oxygen to relieve breathlessness and bluish cast to lips, medication to ease chest pain, and in the case of mycoplasma, some relief from the violent cough—anything that can produce and maintain in the patient the best possible conditions for recovery.

Don't Rush Your Recovery!

The vigorous young person may lead a normal life within a week of his [or her] recovery from pneumonia. For the middle-aged, however, weeks may elapse before they regain their accustomed strength, vigor, and feeling of well being. A person should not be discouraged from returning to work or carrying out usual activities, but must be warned to expect some difficulties. Adequate rest is important to maintain progress toward full recovery and to avoid relapse.

Prevention Is Possible

Because pneumonia is a common complication of influenza (flu), getting a flu shot every fall is good pneumonia prevention.

Vaccine is also available to help fight pneumococcal pneumonia—*one type* of bacterial pneumonia. Your doctor can help you decide if you—or a member of your family—needs the vaccine against pneumococcal pneumonia. It is usually given only to people at high risk of getting the disease and its life-threatening complications. Ask your doctor if you should be vaccinated. The greatest risk of pneumococcal pneumonia usually is among people who:

- Have chronic illnesses such as lung disease, heart disease, kidney disorders, sickle cell anemia, or diabetes.
- Are recovering from severe illness.
- Are in nursing homes or other chronic care facilities.
- Are age 65 or older.

The vaccine is generally given only once. Ask your doctor about revaccination recommendations. It is not recommended for pregnant women or children under age two.

Since pneumonia often follows ordinary respiratory infections, the most important preventive measure is for a person to be alert to any symptoms of respiratory trouble that linger more than a few days. Good health habits—proper diet and hygiene, plentiful rest, regular exercise, etc.— increase resistance to all respiratory illnesses. They also help promote fast recovery if the illnesses do occur.

If You Have Symptoms Of Pneumonia

1. Call your doctor immediately. Even with the many effective antibiotics, early diagnosis and treatment are important.

2. Follow your doctor's advice. If he [or she] says you should be in the hospital, go there. If he [or she] says you may stay at home if you stay in bed, be sure you **STAY** in bed.

3. To prevent recurrence of pneumonia— continue to take the medicine your doctor prescribes until he [or she] says you may stop.

4. Remember—even though pneumonia can be satisfactorily treated, it is an extremely serious illness.

Source: American Lung Association, 1990.

When this occurs, oxygen/carbon dioxide exchange cannot occur in the affected portion of the lung(s). Symptoms of the disease include the abrupt onset of cough, fever, shortness of breath, and, occasionally, chest discomfort. Pneumonia is usually diagnosed through a combination of evaluating the patient's history, a physical examination, and a chest X ray. Treatment almost always includes the use of antibiotics. Many different organisms can cause pneumonia, including bacteria, viruses, and fungi. Researchers have isolated some bacteria that commonly cause pneumonia and have developed a vaccine with them. People at high risk should obtain this vaccination on advice of their health-care professional. Although the vaccine may not prevent all forms of pneumonia, it can help fight off some of the most common kinds. People with chronic lung disease, such as bronchitis, emphysema, and asthma, are especially at risk and should receive the vaccine.

Chronic lung diseases are a widespread problem in the United States, contributing significantly to personal disability. Smoking is the major environmental irritant causing chronic lung diseases, and the best prevention is to avoid or stop smoking. Other environmental and occupational irritants are known to cause chronic lung diseases. Great care should be taken in the workplace and elsewhere to minimize exposure to these irritants. For those with established lung diseases, a pneumonia vaccination and annual flu immunization may help prevent the acute illnesses that, if contracted, may be life-threatening. ▮

5

Metabolic and Endocrine Disorders

Lipid: A class of fatty substances that are insoluble in water, transported throughout the body by the blood, and are one of the body's important sources of food energy; the more important types of lipids include triglycerides (the principal component of body fat) and sterols such as cholesterol.

Dietary cholesterol: Cholesterol contained in the diet; cholesterol intake.

Blood cholesterol: Cholesterol contained in the blood; blood cholesterol levels vary significantly from person to person and are determined by a complex mixture of factors, including cholesterol intake level and the quantity of cholesterol produced by the body.

DISORDERS OF THE METABOLIC and endocrine systems are often grouped together because the two systems work together to regulate the metabolic balance in the body. Chapter 2 briefly touched on cholesterol disorders, which will be more fully explained here. The chapter will pay special attention to diabetes, an endocrine disorder stemming from pancreatic dysfunction, and will also consider the nature and prevention of osteoporosis, a disorder that results from a calcium deficiency.

HYPERLIPIDEMIA

Hyperlipidemia refers to an elevated cholesterol and **lipid** level in the blood. Studies have shown that consuming a diet high in fat can increase one's risk of suffering coronary artery disease. Scientists suspect that it is a risk factor for cancer as well.

Cholesterol has received significant public attention recently, based primarily on two pieces of data. First, there is a strong correlation between early coronary artery disease and blood cholesterol levels. Second, lowering blood cholesterol reduces the risk for heart disease. That coronary artery disease is the number-one cause of death in the United States makes this data even more significant.

Total **dietary cholesterol** is an important risk factor for death from heart disease. The total amount of fat in the diet directly relates to the **blood cholesterol** level, as do heredity and gender. Of these factors, only diet is modifiable.

What Is Cholesterol?

Cholesterol is a fat-soluble steroid crucial to the proper functioning of animal cells. Its structure is very different from that of **fatty acids**, which are also called fats.

Cholesterol is manufactured by the body, primarily the liver, and obtained from the diet. It travels through the circulatory system in spherical particles called **lipoproteins**, so named because they contain both lipids and proteins. An individual's cholesterol level is determined in part by heredity and in part by the fat and cholesterol content of the diet. Obesity and physical inactivity may also be factors. [1]

According to recent scientific research, blood cholesterol level is more significantly influenced by dietary saturated fats than by dietary cholesterol. [2] Although some studies show that dietary cholesterol does seem to have some influence on death rates from coronary heart disease (a finding implying that dietary cholesterol affects blood cholesterol level to some degree), there is a more direct link between blood cholesterol levels and the amount of fats consumed.

Blood cholesterol measurements include the total amount of all types of blood cholesterol. Not all of this cholesterol, however, is harmful. In fact, researchers and doctors have discovered that there are two different kinds of cholesterol, one harmful and one beneficial. Low-density lipoproteins (**LDL cholesterol**), the harmful type, accumulate in tissues and artery linings. But the beneficial type, high-density lipoproteins (**HDL cholesterol**), actually carry LDL cholesterol *away* from the tissues.

What Are Fats?

To understand fats, we must first understand the way that fatty acid chains, composed primarily of carbon atoms, bond to become either saturated or unsaturated. If every available bond site or "arm" of the carbon atom chain bonds with a hydrogen atom, the fatty acid is termed saturated—filled to capacity with hydrogen atoms. If the fatty acid chain has available bond sites, or empty arms, the fatty acid is termed unsaturated.

Fats fall into three categories:

- **Saturated fats**: These are fatty acid chains containing the maximum possible number of carbon and hydrogen bonds. Commonly called the tropical fats because they are found in coconut oil, palm and palm kernel oil, and cocoa butter, saturated fats are also found in beef. These fats are especially responsible for increasing cholesterol levels. They should be kept to a minimum in a healthy diet.

Fatty acids: Chemical compounds containing carbon, hydrogen, and oxygen. They form part of the triglycerides in food and in the body and can be saturated, polyunsaturated, or monounsaturated.

Lipoproteins: A class of proteins found in the blood that consist of a simple protein combined with a lipid (fatty substances that are otherwise insoluble in water). They are transported throughout the body by the blood.

LDL cholesterol: The so-called bad cholesterol; a form of cholesterol that is deposited on the walls of arteries, contributing to the process of atherosclerosis and thus the risk of heart disease.

HDL cholesterol: The so-called good cholesterol, a lipid compound that contains cholesterol removed from the arteries; high HDL cholesterol levels reduce the risk of heart disease.

Saturated fat: A type of fatty acid containing the maximum possible amount of hydrogen; palm oil, coconut oil, and most animal fats are highly saturated fats.

FIGURE 5.1
LDL and HDL Cholesterol

LDL
(LOW-DENSITY LIPOPROTEIN)

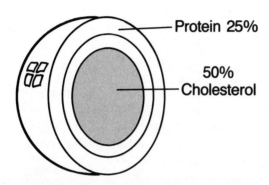

Protein 25%

50%
Cholesterol

HDL
(HIGH-DENSITY LIPOPROTEIN)

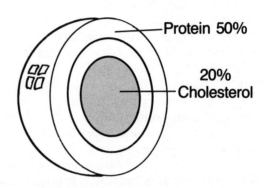

Protein 50%

20%
Cholesterol

Source: Leonard Dank, Medical Illustrations.

LDL (low-density lipoprotein) cholesterol accumulates in the tissues and artery linings. Fifty percent of an LDL molecule is made up of cholesterol. HDL (high-density lipoprotein) cholesterol transports the LDL cholesterol away from the tissues. Fifty percent of an HDL molecule is made up of protein and only 20 percent is cholesterol.

Monounsaturated fats: These are one of two types of unsaturated fats, fats that contain less than the maximum possible amount of hydrogen. Monounsaturated fats contain one less hydrogen bond than the maximum number possible.

Polyunsaturated fats: One of two types of unsaturated fats, fats that contain less than the maximum possible amount of hydrogen. Polyunsaturated fats contain two or more fewer hydrogen bonds than the maximum number possible.

• **Monounsaturated fats**: These are fats that contain one less than the maximum possible number of hydrogen bonds. Fats in this category include olive, canola (rapeseed), and fish oils. Diets that contain proportionately more of these kinds of fats, when compared to the saturated fatty acids, result in lower blood LDL cholesterol levels. These are the best kinds of fats to have in your diet and may safely comprise from 10 to 15 percent of your total calorie intake.
• **Polyunsaturated fats**: These are fatty acid chains that have 2 or more empty bond sites. They are a healthier choice than saturated fats but not as healthy as the monounsaturated oils. Examples of polyunsaturated oils include sunflower and safflower oils.

High Cholesterol
The National Cholesterol Education Program has developed guidelines concerning acceptable blood cholesterol levels. [3]

Table 5.1 Fatty Acid Composition of the Principal Vegetable Oils and Animal Fats*

Did You Know That . . .

Oil or Fat	% of Total Fatty Acids†		
	Saturated	Monoun-saturated	Polyun-saturated
Coconut oil	92	6	2
Palm kernel oil	82	15	2
Butterfat	63	31	3
Cocoa butter	61	34	3
Palm oil	50	40	10
Beef tallow	46	47	4
Lard	42	48	10
Cottonseed oil	26	20	55
Olive oil	17	72	11
Soybean oil	15	24	61
Peanut oil	14	50	32
Corn oil	13	28	59
Sunflower oil	12	19	69
Safflower oil	9	13	78
Low-erucic acid rapeseed oil (canola oil)	6	62	32

Most experts now believe that the relatively high blood cholesterol levels among Americans is in part the result of the American diet, which is higher in fat and cholesterol than that of many other countries.

*Adapted from *Food Fats and Oils.*
†Component fatty acids may not add to 100% because of rounding.

Source: "Typical Fatty Acid Composition of the Principal Vegetable Oils and Animal Fats," *Journal of the American Medical Association,* Vol. 263, No. 5, 2 February 1990, p. 694.

Some popular oils and fats and their fatty acid composition. The healthiest of these choices contain low amounts of saturated fatty acids and high amounts of monoun-saturated fatty acids.

People under the age of 20 should have a blood cholesterol level under 190 mg/dl (milligrams per deciliter). The level for those over the age of 20 should be below 200 mg/dl. In adults, a cholesterol level between 200 and 240 mg/dl is considered borderline.

Specific guidelines are also available for HDL and LDL cholesterol. HDL cholesterol usually measures between 35 and 75 mg/dl. It is inversely related to heart disease, so that the higher the level, the lower the risk for heart disease. Conversely, LDL cholesterol levels are directly related to heart disease, and the lower the reading, the lower the risk for heart disease. Keeping

FIGURE 5.2

**Estimated Percentage of Americans with Serum Cholesterol
of 200 mg/dl or More**

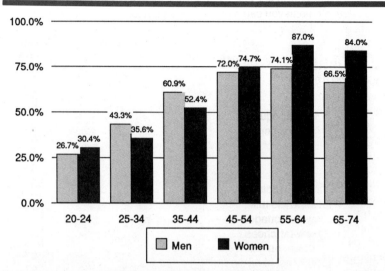

Source: American Heart Association, *1991 Heart and Stroke Facts,* p. 9.

The news is not good. Although the maximum recommended cholesterol level for adults is 200 mg/dl, over 50 percent of Americans above the age of 34 have a cholesterol level exceeding that figure. In women aged 55–64, a staggering 87 percent are considered borderline or at high risk for heart disease.

the LDL cholesterol level below 130 mg/dl is important. An LDL cholesterol of 140 to 150 mg/dl is considered acceptable. A level above 160 mg/dl calls for treatment, especially if other risk factors for heart disease are present.

How Cholesterol Is Checked and When It Should Be Done
Measuring blood cholesterol level involves a simple blood test. Because cholesterol levels can vary from moment to moment, doctors will usually test a person's level 2 or 3 times and then average them. The first of these exams should occur when the patient is 20 years of age and should be repeated every 5 years. People with borderline levels should repeat the test 1 year later. Those with high total blood cholesterol levels should be rechecked every 6 months. Children who come from a family with a strong history of elevated cholesterol levels should begin to have their levels checked as early as age 2.

(continued on p. 116)

1. The heart-healthy diet is not a starvation diet—you can choose from a wide variety of foods, appetizingly prepared. You'll need time to get used to a healthy diet, but most people enjoy it once they do.

2. Meat is a major source of cholesterol and saturated fats, but that doesn't mean you can never eat it. Think of meat as a side dish in a meal, not the centerpiece. Choose lean meats: turkey and chicken breast, lean chops, top round beef. Pork and ham are fine, if you stick to lean cuts. Trim all visible fat. Don't eat poultry skin. Fish is an excellent choice, but not lobster, shrimp, squid, or crab, as they are high in cholesterol. Two 3-ounce or 4-ounce servings of meat or fish a day, or one serving plus two 8-ounce glasses of milk or one cup of cottage cheese will supply all the protein you need.

Tips for a Cholesterol-Lowering Diet

3. Limit or even eliminate whole milk, butter, and other whole-milk products. Don't be fooled by milk labels that say 2% fat. That's almost as much fat as whole milk, which is 3.3% fat by volume. Stick to 1% or skim milk, low-fat cottage cheese, and low-fat or nonfat yogurt. There are no truly low-fat cheeses, so keep portions small.

4. Cut down on all fats. If you want fats for cooking, salad dressings, or homebaked goods, choose unsaturated types. Monoun-saturated fats (olive and canola oil) and polyunsaturated fats (corn and safflower oils, and tub margarines) tend to lower cholesterol. Don't cook with animal fats such as butter or lard. In general, avoid fried foods.

5. Steer clear of fast foods, junk foods, packaged baked goods, and such highly processed foods as luncheon meats, bacon, and sausages, which are almost invariably high in saturated fats (not to mention salt).

6. Add more fruits and vegetables to your daily fare. Try new ones. Serve two or three vegetables at your main meal instead of one. Starchy vegetables, such as potatoes, beans, and winter squash, are very good for you and, contrary to myth, won't cause weight gain if you eat reasonable amounts and forgo the toppings of butter or sour cream.

7. If you like sweets, you can have them. Sugar does not raise cholesterol or do any other harm, except possibly cause cavities and add empty calories. But avoid desserts with potent combinations of sugar, eggs, cream, and butter. Switch from premium ice cream to ice milk, frozen low-fat yogurt, or sherbet.

8. Increase your intake of fiber, particularly the soluble kind (found in beans, oat bran, and rice bran), which has the potential to lower blood cholesterol levels.

9. Unless you never eat meats or whole milk products, you should limit your egg consumption to a total of four a week, remembering that most baked goods contain eggs.

> 10. If you eat frequently in restaurants, apply these same rules to menu choices. Be wary of sauces, gravies, and stews, which may contain hidden fats. Don't hesitate to ask questions about ingredients and preparation methods. If you eat out only rarely, as a treat, you needn't worry so much about what you choose.
>
> 11. Stick with these guidelines every day that you can. But a small treat once in a while won't hurt you.
>
> Source: "Commonsense Tips for a Cholesterol-Lowering Diet—Without Counting Calories or Milligrams," *Johns Hopkins Medical Letter,* January 1990, p. 5.

Influences on HDL Cholesterol Levels

Because HDL cholesterol has a protective effect against heart disease, keeping it as high as possible is a reasonable goal. In general, people who are not overweight and who do not smoke have higher levels of the desirable HDL. Regular exercise increases HDL levels, even after a heart attack. [4] One ounce of alcohol per day has been shown to increase the HDL cholesterol level. However, alcohol may also elevate triglycerides, another form of fat in the blood, so it isn't always beneficial. Furthermore, more than 1 ounce per day increases the risk of cardiovascular disease, including high blood pressure. The female hormone estrogen is thought to elevate HDL cholesterol, which may explain why women have relatively high HDL cholesterol levels and few heart attacks during the years they menstruate regularly.

How to Lower Blood Cholesterol

The majority of people can lower overall blood cholesterol and LDL cholesterol and then maintain a healthy range through diet alone. Cholesterol is found in animal products such as eggs, meat, butter, cheese, and liver or organ meats, items that should be minimized in the diet. Using unsaturated fats is preferable to saturated fats. Fat should comprise 30 percent or less of your total caloric intake.

DIABETES

Insulin: A hormone produced by the pancreas in varying amounts depending on the level of blood sugar; it promotes the absorption and use of glucose by the liver and muscles.

Glucose: A simple sugar that is the major energy source for the cells of the body.

Diabetes is a disorder characterized by a lack of **insulin**, a hormone produced by the pancreas that helps bodily tissue digest **glucose**, a bodily sugar. Ten million Americans, or about 1 in 25 people, have diabetes. It is the seventh leading cause of death in the United States. [5]

(continued on p. 118)

Table 5.2 Count Down on Cholesterol

Type of Food	Cholesterol (mg/dl)	
Apples, oranges, strawberries and all fruits	0	LOW
Bran, whole wheat, oatmeal and all grains	0	
Broccoli, celery, potatoes and all vegetables	0	
Margarine (1 tsp.)	0	
Skim milk (1 cup)	5	
Mayonnaise (2 tsp.)	7	
French fries (1 portion fast food)	9	
Butter (1 tsp.)	11	
1% low-fat milk (1 cup)	14	
Apple pie (1 average slice)	19	
Macaroni & cheese (1 cup)	21	
2% low-fat milk (1 cup)	22	
Hamburger (3½ oz. fast food)	26	
Hard cheese (1 oz.)	30	
Hot dog (2 oz.)	32	
Whole milk (1 cup)	34	
Oysters (3½ oz.)	45	
Tuna, canned (3 oz.)	55	
Porterhouse steak (3½ oz.)	70	
Light-meat chicken or turkey (3½ oz. no skin)	80	
Ice cream (16% fat) (1 cup)	85	
Lobster (3½ oz.)	85	
Cheeseburger (4 oz. fast food)	88	
Dark-meat chicken or turkey (3½ oz. no skin)	95	
Crab (3½ oz.)	100	
Shrimp (3½ oz.)	150	
Egg yolk (1)	270	
Beef liver (3½ oz.)	440	
Beef kidney (3½ oz.)	700	HIGH

Source: National Heart, Lung, and Blood Institute, Department of Health and Human Services, July 1986.

This table lists foods notable for high- or low-cholesterol content. As a rule, dietary cholesterol levels should not exceed 300 milligrams a day.

Did You Know That . . .

Eighty-seven percent of 32,200 adults surveyed in the United States in 1988 knew about the relationship of high cholesterol to heart disease, up from 81 percent in 1986 and 77 percent in 1983.

Diabetes impairs the body's ability to use the fuel it obtains from digestion. Digestion is a process of breaking down and absorbing food in the form of usable molecules, which are then excreted by the body. Glucose is the immediate fuel for most of the body's tissues. But if insulin is not present, glucose cannot be broken down or excreted and remains in the body's bloodstream.

There are 2 kinds of diabetes. Both impair glucose utilization, but the mechanisms are different. Seventy-five to 90 percent of diabetics have adult-onset diabetes, also called Type II or noninsulin-dependent (these 3 terms are used interchangeably). [6] In these people, the pancreas produces insulin, but it seems to have little effect on the blood sugar, a phenomenon called insulin resistance. In Type I diabetes, called insulin-dependent diabetes, the pancreas produces little if any insulin. Those who have this form of diabetes require daily insulin shots for survival.

The Causes of Diabetes

There is no simple answer to the question of what causes diabetes. Type I, or insulin-dependent diabetes, accounts for about 10 percent of all diabetes cases. It usually occurs before the age of 40 and appears to be brought on by a combination of an inherited susceptibility and a viral infection which causes the immune system to mistake the body's insulin-producing cells for a foreign invader and destroy them. Once this occurs, the body can no longer make its own insulin. Type II, or noninsulin-dependent diabetes, appears also to be partially genetic in origin but is also strongly associated with obesity.

Symptoms

Thirst and frequent urination are the most common symptoms of both forms of diabetes. This is because after a meal, the glucose level in the blood rises. If there is no insulin or if it is ineffective, the blood-sugar level remains elevated. The body reacts by increasing urination in an attempt to rid itself of glucose through the urine. The resulting reduction in bodily fluid level triggers a sensation of thirst. Fatigue or a vague ill feeling may also accompany diabetes.

Diagnosis

A normal blood-sugar level is in the range of 60 to 110 mg/dl. A diagnosis of diabetes requires that on 2 testing occasions, this level be greater than 140 mg/dl after an overnight fast or that the blood-sugar level exceed 200 mg/dl 2 hours after a meal. [7]

FIGURE 5.3
The Insulin Infusion Pump

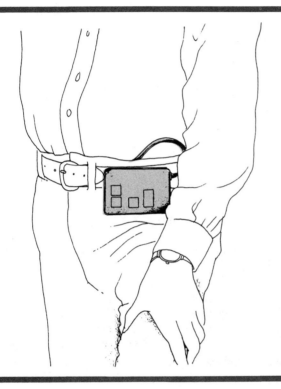

An insulin infusion pump is sometimes recommended for diabetics who need more than one injection of insulin each day in order to control their level. The device is worn around the waist and supplies regulated doses of insulin through a catheter inserted into the abdominal cavity.

Treatment

The best way to treat adult-onset diabetes is through weight reduction, diet, and exercise. Many diabetics are able to control their disease through weight loss alone. The American Diabetes Association recommends a diet in which 50 to 60 percent of total daily calories come from carbohydrates, 12 to 20 percent from protein, and less than 30 percent from fat sources. [8] Doctors recommend a diet that will lead to a gradual weight loss, such as 1 pound per week. The more restrictive diets should never be followed without direct medical supervision. Because diabetics may have elevated blood-lipid levels, watching cholesterol and fat intake is very important.

Did You Know That . . .

The rates of juvenile diabetes are on the rise in New Zealand, Japan, and among African Americans living in the United States. In Finland, where juvenile diabetes was once uncommon, the disease now affects 40 out of 100,000 children annually.

FIGURE 5.4
Testing Blood Sugar Levels

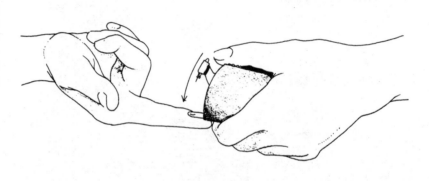

To test glucose levels, a diabetic pricks his or her finger with a special device, similar to the one illustrated here. A drop of blood is then placed on a chemical strip that changes colors depending upon the amount of glucose present.

Exercise has several benefits for diabetics. First, it burns calories, an action that can lessen anyone's total body weight. Second, it heightens the body's response to insulin, so that fewer insulin injections are required to help the body digest glucose.

Type I diabetics require insulin injections. Often, a short-acting and long-acting insulin will be given at the same time. Medications may or may not be necessary to control Type II diabetes. Oral medications used to treat diabetes function primarily to stimulate the pancreas to produce more insulin.

Monitoring Diabetes

The healthy body has a built-in mechanism that keeps the blood sugar in the normal range. When sugar is too high, the body produces more insulin. When blood sugar is too low, the liver releases stored glucose. Diabetics have lost this regulatory mechanism and must check their blood-sugar levels themselves. Many home kits are available to help do this. They allow the diabetic to evaluate the effect of certain foods, exercise, alcohol, and stress on his or her blood-sugar levels. And, although managing diabetes is clearly a team effort involving the patient and the health-care provider, the greater share of the day-to-day responsibilities involved in monitoring and treating diabetes must be borne by the patient.

(continued on p. 122)

Steve Young, 23-year-old printing manager at Young's Printing Co. and Middletown native, was diagnosed with Type-I diabetes at age 2. Here, excerpts from a conversation with him reveal a wonderful attitude and amazing self-discipline that have kept him going for two decades without evidence of diabetic complications.

"I think I've done pretty well with diabetes; my grandfather did just as well, if not better. He was diagnosed as a Type-I diabetic at age 31 and lived until age 83—passing away just a couple of years ago. He worked at Young's for 72 years.

A Healthy Attitude

"From what I've heard, my grandfather was very active and extremely athletic—a great tennis player. He also swam, played golf and did a lot of gymnastics and trapeze work at the Middlesex YMCA. He played almost every sport. He was also very strong: When he was younger, he could walk on his hands up the stairs! He did very well with diabetes, which gave me a good example to follow."

"When I was a kid I never thought diabetes was a problem. The only diabetics I knew were my grandfather and myself, and we didn't have any problems with it. As I grew older, I met other diabetics. Most of them were struggling with it. Even the ones who were really caring for it were struggling—sugar levels too high, too low, always going into reaction, taking several shots a day, testing blood sugar five or six times a day. I wouldn't want to do all that. One shot a day is enough for me."

"I don't know, maybe I'm fortunate. Maybe there are different degrees of diabetes; maybe it's harder to control in some people."

"Because I've had good control over my 21 years as a diabetic, I usually have a good sense of when I need more food and when I need less. I can tell roughly what my sugar level is without testing it by how much I've eaten, what I've done during the day and how I feel. One of the key elements in controlling diabetes is to maintain a consistent day-to-day pattern of life."

"Since I'm more active in the summer, I take a little less insulin than I do in the winter. I also make day-to-day adjustments if needed. If I'm going to play sports all day, I'll take a little less insulin along with a little more food to balance my sugar level with my increased activity level. If I'm going to a dinner party where I might eat a little more than usual, I try to compensate by eating less beforehand, taking a little more insulin or exercising before or after dinner. The most important factor in eating out is to eat and drink the right foods in moderation. To a diabetic, food is a type of medication needed to survive. The right food at the right time in the 'correct dosage' is needed to live a healthy life."

"I was raised by my family to eat good food. When I was little, I'd have candy once in a while. In school, it seemed like everyone was eating it all day long. I'd take a little bit—a corner of a caramel or

Did You Know That . . .

Smoking is particularly risky for people with diabetes. People with diabetes who smoke increase their risk of developing hardening of the arteries (atherosclerosis), which, in turn, restricts blood flow and can greatly increase the risk of kidney disease.

something like that—just to try it. But I never really overdid it. I guess I'm self-disciplined."

"My parents always ate well. We never had junk food in the house. Once in a while we'd have ice cream. I don't think it's because I'm diabetic, I think they would have been that way anyway. My sister never ate much junk food either. We were just brought up that way."

"If all of a sudden there were a cure for diabetes, I still wouldn't eat sweets. I wouldn't change my diet at all."

"If I show too much sugar in my blood, I eat less or I exercise. A lot of times, if I show heavy sugar, I'll just go out and run five miles or something like that."

"Usually I can feel if an insulin reaction is coming on. I'll usually get tired and break into a cold sweat; sometimes I won't really know what's going on—like I'm 'spacing out.' One time I had a reaction at the YMCA; the people there called the ambulance because they thought I was on drugs."

"A lot of people wear those tags that say, 'I am a diabetic.' I don't. But I do carry a card in my wallet now. I guess you really should carry some identification, in case there is a problem. But I try to take care of myself and make sure there won't be any problems. If I'm out by myself or with people who don't understand diabetes, it's always good to play it a little safe, to have a little extra food to make sure I don't go into reaction. You really have to think ahead."

"Tension, I've found, is one of the major things that affects control of diabetes. The amount of stress it puts on your body is like running a marathon. It makes your sugar level drop."

"I think one of the biggest problems young diabetics have is admitting they're diabetic. A lot of them will go to a party and if there is no diet soda, they will pick up a regular soda and drink it. They're embarrassed to say they can't drink it, but they shouldn't be."

"I'd like to help other people learn to control diabetes better. But I think a lot of people never will—unless they change their life-style."

"I think if people could feel today the pains of the complications they might have later, they'd try much harder to control their diabetes."

Source: *Healthline*, Summer 1989, pp. 22–23.

Complications

A key reason for controlling diabetes is to prevent its complications. Heart disease is the most common long-term disease associated with diabetes. Diabetics have twice the risk of heart disease as nondiabetics. Other long-term complications include kidney disease, eye problems, blindness, and nerve damage.

Risk Factors

Type II diabetes is far more common among obese people than among those of normal weight. Why obesity affects the body's ability to use insulin is unknown. It is clear, however, that obesity is an important factor in noninsulin-dependent diabetes. It is not, however, the only risk factor to consider. The likelihood of developing Type II diabetes increases with age. Family medical history plays a role as well; studies show that having a parent or a sibling with Type II diabetes increases one's risk of suffering the same disorder.

OSTEOPOROSIS

Osteoporosis is defined as a loss of bone mass. Loosely translated from its Greek root, it means thinner, more brittle bones. Significant osteoporosis, which leads to fractures, affects 35 percent of women over the age of 60 and is a contributing factor in 700,000 fractures annually. [9]

Cause

The bones in the adult human are in a continuous state of formation and breakdown. When osteoporosis occurs, there is a prolonged imbalance between the rate of bone formation and **resorption,** the breakdown phase. The reason this imbalance occurs is unknown. Male and female hormones, calcium, vitamin D, and **parathyroid hormone,** secreted in a gland next to the thyroid, all play a part in regulating bone formation and resorption.

The bones most commonly affected by osteoporosis are near the hip, the wrist, and the spine. Affected women begin losing bone density around the age of 30 to 35. The loss increases at menopause.

Symptoms and Diagnosis

Unless a fracture occurs, osteoporosis does not have definite symptoms. The most common fractures occur at the hip, just above the wrist, and in the back. The typical slouching figure of an aging woman may be accounted for by repeated fractures of the vertebrae collapsing upon themselves.

Aside from a fracture, the only way to diagnose osteoporosis is through a test that measures bone density. It is not always accurate, however, and doctors rarely perform it. X rays may show some sign of aging or brittle bones but often will show

Osteoporosis: A disturbance of bone metabolism in which the bone mass decreases and the bones become more fragile.

Resorption: The organic breaking down of a structure into parts and the assimilation of those parts for a different use.

Parathyroid hormone: A hormone produced by the parathyroid glands, located in the neck, that helps to control the level of calcium in the blood.

FIGURE 5.5
Progressive Spinal Deformity in Osteoporosis

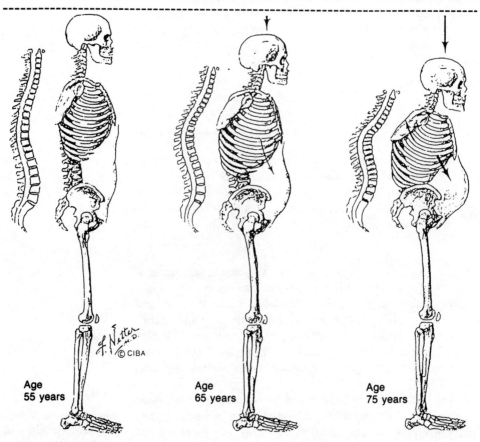

Age
55 years

Age
65 years

Age
75 years

Source: F. Kaplan, *Clinical Symposia CIBA* 35, No. 5, 1983.

Fractures of the vertabrae are common in cases of osteoporosis. These fractures compress over the years and may lead to loss of height, a distended abdomen, and the typical dowager's hump.

nothing even after 30 percent of the bone mass has been lost. [10] Calcium levels in the blood are usually normal.

Prevention and Treatment
Prevention again means minimizing the risk factors. If you smoke, stop. Eat a diet that is high in calcium. Foods rich in calcium include collard greens, broccoli, oysters, salmon, sar-

Table 5.3 Top 10 Calcium-Rich Foods

Food	Serving Size	Calcium (mg)	Calories
Sardines (canned in oil, drained solids with bones)	3¹/₄ oz	402	187
Swiss cheese (low-fat)	1 oz	345	84
Ricotta cheese (part-skim)	¹/₂ cup	337	171
Collards, frozen	1 cup	299	51
Milk (skim)	1 cup	296	88
Yogurt (plain, lowfat)	8 oz	271	113
Salmon, pink (canned, including bones)	3 oz	215	155
Broccoli	1 medium stalk	158	47
Kale, frozen, cooked and drained	1 cup	157	40
Tofu	4 oz	145	82

Nutrient and calorie information based on U.S. Department of Agriculture Handbooks # 456 and 8–1.

Source: *Redbook,* March 1989, p. 22.

Including more calcium in the diet is a good way to avoid osteoporosis. Here is a list of some calcium-rich foods.

dines, and most dairy products. Exercise increases the stress on bones and stimulates bone formation. Administration of post-menopausal estrogens should be an option for women, especially those at high risk of developing osteoporosis.

Although there is no definite treatment for osteoporosis, physicians have prescribed estrogen therapy for some patients because this hormone has been found to decrease the rate at which bone is lost. Often this therapy will be combined with calcium supplements to strengthen bones more dramatically.

The Risk of Cancer Associated with Estrogens

Estrogen therapy has proven beneficial in treating osteoporosis, in possibly helping to protect against the risk of cardiovascular disease, and in diminishing hot flashes associated with menopause. However, studies have shown that prolonged estrogen treatment increases the risk of cancer of the uterus. To diminish the risk of cancer in those women who would benefit from its use,

(continued on p. 127)

At least one-third of all women over 50 in the U.S. and nearly one-half of all women past 75 suffer from osteoporosis, according to the National Osteoporosis Foundation. Caused by a gradual deterioration of skeletal tissue, osteoporosis can make bones so weak that even a minor fall or a friendly hug can break them. "Crush fractures" of the spinal column also may result and can trigger back pain, cause a decrease in height and create a humped back. How can you prevent osteoporosis? One major strategy: Get plenty of calcium in your diet every day.

Keeping Bones Straight and Strong

The number-one bone food

Your body stores about 99 percent of its calcium in bones and teeth. The rest, found in blood and other tissues, helps muscles contract and blood to pump and clot. When your diet is low in calcium, your body "steals" from your bones, placing the skeleton in jeopardy, cautions William A. Peck, M.D., president of the National Osteoporosis Foundation and author of *Osteoporosis: The Silent Thief* (Scott Foresman, 1988).

And as you grow older things can get worse. After age 35, bone-tissue loss exceeds bone replacement and the skeletal structure becomes less dense. "Adding extra calcium to your diet once bone depletion has occurred can protect what's left, but it won't restore lost bone," stresses Robert P. Heaney, M.D., professor of endocrinology at Creighton University in Omaha, Nebraska, and author of *Calcium and Common Sense* (Doubleday, 1988). "The key is to build up the optimum amount of bone mass before this decline begins."

How much do you need?

The Recommended Dietary Allowance (RDA) of calcium for women and men over 18 is 800 milligrams daily (less than the amount contained in about three 8-ounce glasses of low-fat milk). More is required during pregnancy. Most experts believe the RDA should be even higher—1,000 milligrams a day for premenopausal women; as much as 1,500 milligrams for postmenopausal women and those in high-risk groups.

But recent studies show that women ages 25 to 74 get only half the RDA. Women are, however, six to eight times more likely than men to develop osteoporosis, because their bones are less dense and their calcium reserves lower. Women also lose calcium during pregnancy, childbirth and after menopause, due to declining levels of the hormone estrogen, which helps prevent bone loss.

How to up your intake

To get more calcium into your diet:

• Add nonfat milk powder to gravies, soups and stews; sprinkle grated low-fat cheese on salads and pasta. Choose vitamin D-enriched milk to increase calcium absorption.

- Eat plenty of fruits and cabbage-family vegetables—both contain the calcium-retaining nutrients boron and vitamin K.
- Stir a teaspoon of vinegar or lemon juice into soups and stews made with bones; also squeeze lemon juice on broccoli and other calcium-rich vegetables: The acid draws out calcium and helps your body absorb it more readily.
- Cut back on fat and protein, which may impede calcium absorption.
- Cut back on caffeine and salt; they step up calcium loss.

Boning up on supplements

If you opt for a supplement, choose one with no more than 100 percent of the RDA. (Exceeding the recommended levels can hinder the absorption of iron and other minerals and increase the risk of kidney stones.) Calcium carbonate tablets are better bets than calcium lactate or gluconate tablets because they're generally smaller, easier to swallow and contain calcium in its most concentrated form. Bypass bone meal or dolomite—some sources are lead-contaminated.

Note: Some calcium supplement brands aren't absorbed as well as others. To test: Drop a tablet in a few ounces of room-temperature vinegar and stir every five minutes or so. If the tablet remains intact beyond 30 minutes, your body won't be able to absorb it.

Are you at risk?

Along with a calcium deficiency, other factors increase your susceptibility to osteoporosis: *Genetics:* Small-boned, fair-skinned women of Caucasian (especially Northern European) or Asian extraction seem most prone. *Early menopause:* When a woman's ovaries stop producing estrogen, she loses its bone-protecting effect. *Lack of exercise:* Without some weight-bearing activities like walking, jogging and skipping rope, bone loss can escalate. *Medications:* Frequent use of certain drugs such as corticosteroids, antacids containing aluminum and some diuretics can "drain" away calcium. Other possible risk factors: *Family history of osteoporosis. Smoking cigarettes and/or excessive alcohol use*—both habits are toxic to bone cells.

Source: *Redbook*, March 1989, p. 22.

Did You Know That . . .

O steoporosis is caused by the slowing down of the normal process of bone-cell replacement in the aging body, and is most likely to occur in people in their 60s, 70s, and 80s.

---

physicians usually combine 2 female hormones, estrogen and progesterone, to mimic the normal monthly menstrual cycle. The estrogen stimulates the cells in the lining of the uterus, and the progesterone allows those cells to mature without impairing estrogen's therapeutic effects on the rest of the body. Long-term studies show that progesterone helps to protect against cancer for those women on estrogen. [11] Typically, a doctor will advise the patient to take estrogen from the 1st through the 15th of each month, to take progesterone from the 16th through the 25th of each month, and then to abstain from both hormones until the first day of the next month, when the cycle begins again.

Risk Factors

Those at highest risk of suffering osteoporosis are women of postmenopausal age. Eating a diet consistently low in calcium may also contribute to the development of osteoporosis. Other risk factors include smoking and heredity (osteoporosis seems to run in families).

Abnormalities of glucose, fat, and calcium metabolism are all significant risk factors for developing chronic disease. The best way to prevent or to control these conditions is to eat a healthful, nutritious diet and to exercise regularly.

A Personal Plan of Action

THE THOUGHT OF MAJOR CHRONIC DISEASES, their risk factors, and their potential consequences can be depressing. It need not be, however. Americans born today are living longer than at any time in history. The average lifespan for a female born in 1990 is 79 years. For males, it is 72 years. [1] The major factor contributing to that longevity is a healthy life-style, and that is under your control. Such a life-style is not only good in its own right, but it prevents or delays the onset of chronic disease—and it helps make those later years happy and healthy.

The key to preventing or delaying the onset of chronic diseases lies first in understanding what causes each disease and what increases the likelihood of developing it. Once you are aware of these facts, you can alter your life-style to minimize your risks.

At this point, you may be wondering just how complicated it is to devise a plan that will help to prevent all or most of the major chronic diseases. At first glance, this may seem an extremely formidable task. Fortunately, there is no need to construct a different plan for each individual disease. Instead, simply follow these 5 basic rules:

- Maintain a well-balanced, low-fat diet.
- Maintain your proper weight.
- Get regular exercise.
- Stop smoking.
- Get regular medical checkups.

Each of these deserves a closer look.

FIGURE 6.1

Life Expectancy at Birth, According to Race and Sex in the United States

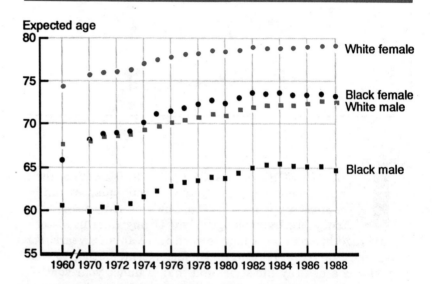

Source: National Center for Health Statistics, National Vital Statistics System.

In 1988, life expectancy at birth was 64.9 years for black males, 72.3 years for white males, 73.4 years for black females, and 78.9 years for white females.

DIET

According to Edwin Bierman, M.D., Professor of Medicine at the University of Washington School of Medicine, "Nutrition is the cornerstone of preventive medicine. In fact, 5 of the 10 leading causes of death in the United States are associated with diet. And the 5 diseases, heart disease, cancer, cerebrovascular disease (stroke), diabetes . . . , and atherosclerosis, are together responsible for nearly 70 percent of all deaths in this country. Three other leading causes of mortality—accidents, suicide, and chronic liver disease—are linked to excessive alcohol consumption." [2]

In short, a proper diet can help prevent heart disease, cancer, and diabetes simultaneously. Dietary recommendations for preventing most diseases overlap nicely, allowing us to draw up basic guidelines. We will look at four aspects of the diet: fat/cholesterol, fiber, calcium, and vitamins.

FIGURE 6.2
Healthy Foods

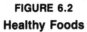
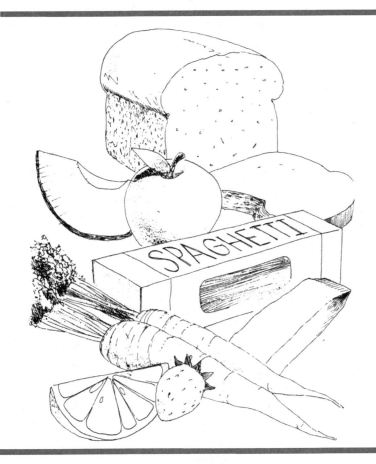

A healthy diet contains a limited amount of fat, sugar, and cholesterol, and includes
daily servings of fresh fruit, vegetables, cereals, breads, and legumes.

Fat and Cholesterol

The recommendations for both preventing and treating high
cholesterol levels are the same. They were outlined in chapter 5
and are summarized here:

1. Consume less than 300 mg of cholesterol per day.

2. Consume less than 30 percent of your total daily calories
   from fats.

3. Consume less than 10 percent of your total daily calories from saturated fats.

For most people, these recommendations mean modifying their diets. Easy modifications include substituting fish, low-fat or nonfat dairy products, skinless poultry, and lean meats for foods higher in fat; consuming more whole grain food products, such as whole wheat bread, cereal, and pasta, instead of high-fat foods; and minimizing or avoiding high-fat foods such as egg yolks, organ meats, and butter. [3]

Fiber, Calcium, and Vitamins
Fiber proponents believe that dietary fiber confers several benefits, from preventing constipation and hemorrhoids to staving off cancer of the colon. [4] The National Cancer Institute recommends eating 20 to 30 grams of fiber per day as a cancer preventive measure. [5] Good sources of fiber are vegetables, fruits, and whole grain cereals.

As mentioned in chapter 5, calcium is another important dietary staple. Women need to be especially conscious of their calcium consumption. A pre-menopausal woman should consume 1,000 mg of calcium per day. A post-menopausal woman should consume about 1,500 mg of calcium per day, provided medical **contraindications**, such as kidney stones or **hypercalcemia**, are not present. Experts recommend foods high in calcium—such as low-fat dairy products (skim milk and yogurt), turnip and collard greens, broccoli, tofu, oysters, sardines, and salmon—over calcium supplement tablets. Of the calcium supplements, calcium carbonate not only has the highest percentage of calcium, but it is also the least expensive. [6] Finally, make sure your diet includes an adequate supply of all vitamins and minerals. Here are some further guidelines for a healthy diet:

- 6 or more servings of cereals/breads/pasta/legumes per day
- 5 or more servings of vegetables and fruits per day
- 4 to 6 one-ounce servings of meat, fish, or protein per day
- 3 to 4 servings of nonfat or low-fat dairy products per day.

Contraindications: Factors in a person's physical condition that make it unwise to pursue a certain line of treatment.

Hypercalcemia: An abnormally high level of calcium in the blood.

WEIGHT CONTROL

Experts estimate that 25 percent of Americans are overweight. [7] Obesity contributes to hypertension, adult-onset diabetes, and

(continued on p. 135)

Table 6.1 Fiber Content of Selected Foods

Item	Serving Size	Dietary Fiber (grams)
BREAD		
whole-wheat, stone-ground	2 slices	2.8
French	2 slices	2.0
pumpernickel	2 slices	8.6
rye	2 slices	1.8
corn, whole-ground	2 pieces	5.4
white, enriched	2 slices	1.0
BREAKFAST CEREALS		
all bran	1/3 cup	10.0
oat flakes	1 cup	4.1
corn bran	3/4 cup	5.9
oat bran	1/3 cup	4.2
shredded wheat, sm.	2/3 cup	3.3
40% branflakes	2/3 cup	4.0
raisin bran	2/3 cup	3.6
bran squares	2/3 cup	5.7
oatmeal, cooked	3/4 cup	2.8
FRUIT		
figs, dried	1 medium	3.7
pear	1 medium	5.0
blackberries	1/2 cup	4.5
dates	2 fruit	1.6
orange	1 small	1.2
raspberries	1/2 cup	4.6
prunes	1/3 cup	5.8
apple with skin	1 fruit	2.8
strawberries	3/4 cup	2.0
cantaloupe	1/2 melon	3.2
raisins	1 1/2 tablespoons	1.0
banana	1 medium	2.0
plums	3 small	1.8
blueberries	1/2 cup	2.5
apricots	2 fruit	1.5
GRAINS		
barley, pearled	2 tablespoons	3.0
cornmeal, whole grain	2 tablespoons	2.3
flour, all-purpose	2 1/2 tablespoons	0.7
flour, dark rye	2 1/2 tablespoons	2.5
flour, whole meal wheat	2 1/2 tablespoons	1.8
oats, rolled, dry	1/3 cup	2.7

(table continues on next page)

Did You Know That . . .

Rather than relying on dieting, most experts recommend that people exercise regularly and eat smaller portions of low-fat, high-fiber meals in order to maintain or reduce body weight.

Item	Serving Size	Dietary Fiber (grams)
LEGUMES		
kidney beans, cooked	1/2 cup	5.8
pinto beans, cooked	1/2 cup	5.3
lima beans, cooked	1/2 cup	4.4
white beans, cooked	1/2 cup	5.0
chick peas	1/2 cup	15.0
green peas, cooked	1/2 cup	4.1
lentils, cooked	1/2 cup	2.0
NUTS AND SEEDS		
almonds, roasted	6 nuts	1.1
peanuts, roasted	10 nuts	0.8
pecans	2 nuts	0.5
walnuts	2 nuts	0.4
RICE, PASTA		
spaghetti	1/2 cup	0.8
rice, brown	1/2 cup	2.4
SNACKS		
crackers, graham	2 squares	2.8
crackers, whole wheat	5 crackers	1.9
VEGETABLES		
asparagus	3/4 cup	3.1
green beans	1/2 cup	2.1
yellow beans	1/2 cup	2.3
broccoli	1/2 cup	2.5
brussels sprouts	1/2 cup	3.9
carrots	1/2 cup	1.3
cauliflower	1/2 cup	2.0
corn	1/2 cup	3.5
eggplant	1/2 cup	2.0
okra	1/2 cup	3.0
parsnips	1/2 cup	3.1
pumpkin, canned	3/4 cup	3.3
sauerkraut, canned	1/2 cup	2.4
spinach	1/2 cup	2.0
acorn squash	1/2 cup	3.6
sweet potato	1 large	3.4
zucchini	1/2 cup	2.7

A chart depicting the fiber levels of various foods. The National Research Council recommends that adults consume about 20 to 30 grams of fiber each day.

elevated blood lipid levels, and it is a risk factor for certain cancers. Obviously, keeping weight under control is one of the best preventive measures you can take to avoid major chronic diseases.

Consuming about 10 calories per pound of current body weight is a good rule of thumb if you are trying to lose weight. The weight will come off more slowly than it would with a more restrictive, "quick-fix" diet, but there is a greater chance that once the weight is off, it will not return. [8]

EXERCISE

Lack of regular exercise is thought to be a risk factor in the development of both heart disease and hypertension. It may also be a risk factor for obesity, noninsulin-dependent diabetes, and osteoporosis.

There is no one "ideal" level or kind of exercise. It varies from person to person, so those who wish to begin an exercise program

The Physical Activity Readiness Questionnaire

1. Has your doctor ever said you have heart trouble?

2. Do you frequently have pains in your heart and chest?

3. Do you often feel faint or have spells of severe dizziness?

4. Has a doctor ever said your blood pressure was too high?

5. Has your doctor ever told you that you have a bone or joint problem, such as arthritis, that has been aggravated by exercise or might be made worse by exercise?

6. Is there a good physical reason not mentioned here why you should not follow an activity program even if you wanted to?

7. Are you over age 65 and not accustomed to vigorous exercise?

If your answer to one or more of these is "yes," see a doctor before beginning any exercise program.

Source: "Physical Activity Readiness," *British Columbia Medical Journal*, Vol. 17, 1975, pp. 375–378.

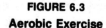

FIGURE 6.3
Aerobic Exercise

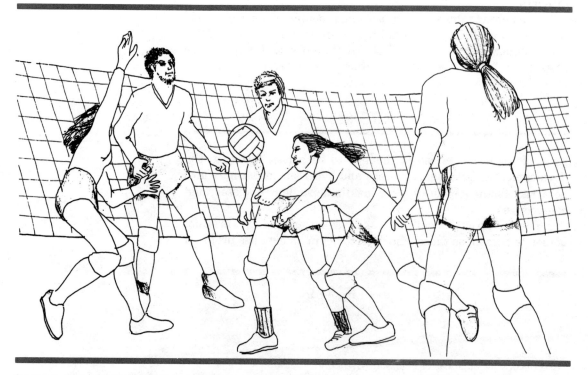

A team sport such as volleyball is an excellent component of a regular aerobic exercise program.

may want to consult with a health-care professional to devise the best possible plan. In addition, doctors cannot determine the exact amount of exercise one would need to prevent all diseases. Generally, they advise their patients to begin with a low-intensity exercise plan, which patients should follow on a regular basis. The intensity and duration of this exercise regimen should increase gradually over a period of months.

Generally, the most healthful exercises are the aerobic ones because they help strengthen the heart and increase its efficiency. Walking is an ideal aerobic activity that is convenient, sociable, and affordable, and it doesn't require special equipment or training. A good short-term goal is to walk for 30 minutes 3 times a week. This may be increased to 30 minutes each day several months later. Fifteen to 45 minutes of vigorous aerobic exercise, 2 to 4 times a week, provides the maximum benefit to

(continued on p. 138)

You ride 4 times a week for a total of 7 hours. A friend cycles 6 times a week and logs 10 hours. Who is improving their fitness more?

The answer is not as simple as it seems. In fact, the question lacks some crucial information—namely, riding intensity.

The 3 most important variables in training are frequency, duration, and intensity. The first 2 are easily monitored, but the third can be elusive.

Target Heart Rate

To determine it, you must know the amount of power you're generating compared to the maximum level you could produce if you were working as hard as possible.

Fortunately, you have a built-in intensity monitor that naturally reports this information. It's your heart rate. It ranges from some minimum value when you're resting to a maximum level during extreme efforts. When riding, your heart rate is at a certain percentage of its maximum. This percentage accurately reflects your exercise intensity. For instance, if your heart rate is at 80% of maximum, you're riding at 80% intensity.

In the 1950s, researchers discovered that to significantly increase fitness you must maintain an intensity level of at least 65%. This value became known as target heart rate. Three decades later, the concept remains the same. To increase your fitness level, your training must hit this physiological bull's-eye.

How can I determine my target heart rate? First, you need to find your maximum heart rate. The most accurate way to do this is by taking a laboratory stress test. However, this is expensive and not essential for recreational cyclists.

An alternative is to estimate your maximum heart rate by subtracting your age from 220. Then, multiply the result by 0.65 and 0.85 to determine your target heart rate zone. For instance, if you're 30 years old, your age-predicted max heart rate is 190 beats per minute (220 − 30). Your target range is 124 (190 × 0.65) to 162 (190 × 0.85) bpm. Whenever you're in this zone—no matter what the exercise—you're training intensely enough to improve cardiovascular fitness. The closer you are to the top of this range, the more benefits you derive.

What's the best way to monitor my heart rate? During a ride, there are several ways to check heart rate. You can monitor your pulse at the carotid artery in your neck (just beside the Adam's apple), or you can check the radial artery in your wrist (at the base of either thumb).

Using your index and middle fingers, count the number of beats in 6 seconds and simply add a zero. Or, to be more accurate, count the number of beats in 15 seconds and multiply by 4.

It'll take practice before you're able to monitor your pulse quickly and easily while riding. Always make sure the road is clear, and don't slow down because your heart rate will too.

To simplify things, there are a number of electronic pulse monitors on the market. These devices typically include a transmitter that straps to the chest and a receiver that fastens around the wrist like a watch. A tiny electrode communicates wirelessly with the receiver, and heart rate readings are displayed.

Good pulse monitors, priced from $125, are accurate and allow heart rate to be tracked throughout a ride. Some models can even interface with computers and generate heart rate graphs.

Is it a waste of time to train below my target heart rate? If you're in good shape, training below your target zone won't improve cardiovascular fitness. However, any exercise is better than no exercise, and going for an occasional easy spin will aid muscle recovery and refresh you mentally.

If you're out of shape, any training brings aerobic improvement.

Isn't it true that I burn more fat at a lower heart rate? Not really. At lower intensities, fat does provide a high percentage of fuel. But overall, you can burn more total fat calories by riding harder.

For example, cycling for one hour at a heart rate of 120 bpm may burn 350 calories. Of these, about half (175) might be fat calories. Conversely, if you pedal harder and get your heart rate to 160 bpm, you might burn 1,000 calories in an hour. At this intensity, only about $1/5$ will be fat calories, but that's still 25 more (200) than the low-intensity ride. So overall, at the higher intensity you burn slightly more fat calories and nearly 3 times as many total calories.

This is doubly significant because of the way our bodies restock used calories. When you ride below your target zone and burn a high percentage of fat calories, your body will replenish these first. Thus, you're back where you started. For losing weight, it's best to ride at the highest level that's comfortably sustainable. Don't restrict your riding intensity in an attempt to burn more fat.

What happens when I train above my target heart rate? Evidence generally indicates that the more intensely you train, the more you'll improve. However, it's unknown whether you can reach a point of diminishing returns. Some experts have suggested that 90% should be the limit for training intensity. But this has yet to be shown scientifically. Most experts agree that a target range between 65% and 85% of maximum is safe and effective. If you routinely ride in this target zone, it's guaranteed you'll become fitter.

Source: Steve Johnson, *Bicycling* (July 1989), p. 81.

Maximum heart rate: The number obtained by subtracting your age from 220; the resulting difference is defined as the maximum heart rate (in number of beats per minute) and should not be exceeded.

the cardiovascular system and is the goal for which you should eventually strive. This will assist you in achieving a sustained heart rate between 65 and 90 percent of your **maximum heart rate**. Maximum heart rate is determined by subtracting your age from 220. [9] Other aerobic activities include jogging, bicycling, swimming, tennis, dancing, aerobic exercise, and basketball.

Table 6.2 Energy Expenditure of Various Physical Activities

Activity	Energy Expenditure: Calories per 30 Minutes
Badminton	147–285
Basketball	207–405
Canoeing	66–129
Climbing hills	183–357
Cycling	
5.5 mph	96–189
9.4 mph	150–294
Dancing, ballroom	78–150
Fishing	93–183
Gardening	
Mowing	168–330
Raking	81–159
Weeding	108–213
Golf	129–249
Running	
11.5 minutes per mile	204–399
9.0 minutes per mile	291–567
Swimming	
Crawl, slow	192–375
Crawl, fast	234–459
Tennis	165–321
Walking, comfortable pace	120–234

Source: Sally S. Harris, "Exercise and the Heart: Report of the U.S. Preventive Services Task Force," *Primary Cardiology,* Vol. 16, No. 3 (March 1990), pp. 41–50.

Some exercises and the calories they burn. Note that walking, an accessible and inexpensive activity, can use as many calories as some of the more strenuous sports.

Did You Know That . . .

Pushing a manual lawnmower burns between 420 and 480 calories an hour, nearly as many as an hour of tennis. This is believed to be one reason that lawnmower sales have more than doubled in recent years.

SMOKING CESSATION

Of all the controllable risk factors for chronic diseases, the most dangerous is smoking. Quitting this habit is the most important step a person can take to prevent the onset of chronic diseases. The American Cancer Society has a "Fresh Start" program to help people quit. Your local American Cancer Society or American Lung Association office or a nearby hospital often will have information about this and other programs available in your area. The American Cancer Society's tips on quitting include:

1. Smoke one fewer cigarette each day.

2. Make smoking each cigarette a special decision and put off making the decision.

3. Don't give up cigarettes "completely." Instead, carry one with you in case of need. Eventually, you'll be saving it for later, permanently.

4. Don't quit "forever." Just stop for a day. And tomorrow try it for another day. And tomorrow and tomorrow.

5. Tell your friends and family you're quitting. A public commitment bolsters willpower.

6. Pick Q (for "Quit") Day and just quit.

7. Destroy evidence of cigarettes—ashtrays, matches, and the like—so you aren't reminded of your renunciation.

8. Carry a supply of chewing gum, cough drops, carrot sticks, and so on. Use them as healthy substitutes.

9. Nervousness and hunger are signs that the body is readjusting. They usually only last a few days or at most a couple of weeks. If they are hard for you to manage, ask your doctor for help. [10]

MEDICAL CHECKUPS

There are many conditions that cause serious illness, disability, and premature death if left untreated. At the same time, medical studies have shown that early diagnosis and treatment can significantly improve the prognosis for individuals with these conditions. The United States Preventive Services Task Force recently listed the best screening devices for chronic diseases. These guidelines complement the American Cancer Society's recommendations for a periodic cancer-related checkup but do not include all of the American Cancer Society's procedures.

These basic recommendations do not apply to those at high risk. If you have significant risk factors for particular diseases, you may want to review the relevant material in this book for guidelines and discuss your situation with a health-care profes-

FIGURE 6.4
Doctor-Patient Consultation

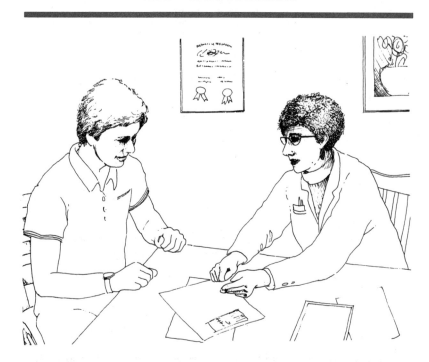

Periodic medical checkups can play a significant role in the early diagnosis of illness.

sional. In addition, if you suffer any symptoms of a major illness, consult your doctor immediately.

The United States Preventive Services Task Force has devised guidelines to help doctors, physician-assistants, and nurse-practitioners establish priorities for preventive health care. However, you may also benefit from this information because it identifies the procedures and tests thought to be most useful for detecting the statistically most important preventable diseases in given age groups. Remember, however, that each individual has a unique heredity and environment. These guidelines are general recommendations; they do not fit every specific situation.

The best way to prevent or minimize chronic disease is to practice good health habits. Follow a well balanced, low-fat, low-

(continued on p. 143)

Physical Examinations

AGES 13–18: (One exam during this time)

1. Leading causes of death: motor vehicle crashes, homicide, suicide, injuries (non-motor vehicle), and heart disease.

2. Screening: dietary intake, physical activity, tobacco/alcohol/drug use, sexual practices.

3. Exam: height, weight, blood pressure.

4. Immunization: diphtheria-tetanus booster.

5. Counseling: diet and exercise, substance use, sexual practices, injury prevention, dental health.

AGES 19–39: (Exam every 1–3 years)

1. Leading causes of death: motor vehicle crashes, homicide, suicide, non-motor vehicle accidental injuries, and heart disease.

2. Screening: dietary intake, physical activity, tobacco/alcohol/drugs, sexual practices.

3. Exam: height, weight, blood pressure.

4. Immunizations: diphtheria-tetanus (every 5–10 years).

5. Lab: non-fasting cholesterol (every 5 years), Pap smear (every 1–3 years).

6. Counseling: diet and exercise, substance use, sexual practices, injury prevention, dental health.

AGES 40–64: (Every 1–3 years)

1. Leading causes of death: heart disease, lung cancer, stroke, breast cancer, colorectal cancer, obstructive lung disease.

2. Screening: dietary intake, physical activity, tobacco/alcohol/drugs, sexual practices.

3. Exam: height, weight, blood pressure, breast (every year).

4. Immunizations: diphtheria-tetanus booster (every 5–10 years).

5. Lab: non-fasting total blood cholesterol, Pap smear, mammogram (every 1–2 years after age 50).

6. Counseling: diet and exercise, substance abuse, sexual practices, injury prevention, dental health.

AGES 65 and older: (Every year)

1. Leading causes of death: heart disease, stroke, chronic obstructive lung disease, pneumonia and/or influenza, lung cancer, and colorectal cancer.

2. Screening: symptoms of prior stroke-like symptoms, diet, physical activity, tobacco/alcohol/drugs, functional status at home.

3. Exam: height, weight, blood pressure, visual acuity, hearing, breast exam.

4. Immunizations: diphtheria-tetanus, flu shot, pneumonia shot.

5. Lab: non-fasting total blood cholesterol, urine sample (dipstick), mammogram, thyroid function.

6. Counseling: diet and exercise, substance abuse, injury prevention, dental health, glaucoma testing.

Source: Adapted from United States Preventive Services Task Force guidelines.

cholesterol diet rich in fiber, calcium and other minerals, and vitamins. Exercise regularly. Conduct self-examinations of your skin and breasts or genitals on a monthly basis. Get regular medical checkups that test blood pressure and cholesterol levels. Following this advice is not difficult and is certainly worthwhile, for it can make your life healthier, happier, and longer. W

Answer Key to "Your Heart and How It Works" Puzzle (Page 4)

ACROSS

2. mitral
3. muscle
6. vein
8. fist
10. valves
12. pump
14. myocardium
16. atrium
17. lung
18. endocardium
19. dioxide
20. arm
21. artery

DOWN

1. aortic
4. pulmonary
5. tissue
6. ventricle
7. pericardium
9. septum
11. tricuspid
13. pulmonary
15. blood
16. aorta

Glossary

A

ACE inhibitor: Medication that inhibits the action of a specific enzyme and thereby blocks one of the stages in a chain of biochemical reactions controlling blood pressure. ACE inhibitors are used to treat hypertension and heart failure.

Aerobic exercise: A form of exercise that increases respiration, intake of oxygen, heart rate, and cardiovascular fitness.

Alveoli: The small air sacs of the lung, where the blood exchanges carbon dioxide for oxygen.

Aneurysm: A weakening of an artery wall.

Angina pectoris: The medical term for chest pain caused by an insufficient supply of oxygen to the heart muscle.

Anticholinergic drugs: A group of drugs that block the action of acetylcholine, a neurotransmitter that stimulates cell activity, thus relieving a range of symptoms, including excessive contraction of the bronchioles associated with asthma.

Antitrypsin enzyme deficiency: A deficiency in the lungs of a chemical known as alpha$_1$-antitrypsin that is thought to protect the lung tissue against emphysema; this deficiency appears to be genetic in origin.

Arrhythmia: Abnormality of heart rhythm.

Arteries: Blood vessels carrying oxygenated blood away from the heart toward the tissues.

Asthma: An abrupt or chronic condition characterized by narrowed airways within the lungs, which causes obstruction of the airflow.

Atherosclerosis: Buildup of cholesterol, fat, and cellular debris within the lining of arteries.

Atrium: Receiving chamber in the heart.

B

Bacterial endocarditis: Infection in the lining of the heart and the heart valves.

Bacterial pneumonia: An inflammation of the lungs caused by bacterial infection; the major symptoms of pneumonia include fever, chills, shortness of breath, and, in more severe cases, the coughing up of sputum or blood.

Balloon angioplasty: Dilating a narrowed artery with a balloon attached to a catheter.

Barium enema: A process in which barium sulfate, a chemical that is visible on X rays, is introduced into the bowel so that the lining of the colon and rectum can be examined by X ray.

Basal cell cancer (carcinoma): The most common and least dangerous form of skin cancer; basal cell cancers originate in the basal layer of the skin; they grow slowly and seldom spread to other areas of the body.

Benign: The opposite of malignant; a tumor that is usually encapsulated, does not infiltrate normal tissue, and does not metastasize.

Beta-blockers: Drugs that simultaneously decrease the heart's rate and contraction strength and increase bronchial muscle tone.

Biopsy: Removal and microscopic examination of tissue from a living body, most frequently from a tumor, for the purpose of determining whether or not it is malignant.

Blood cholesterol: Cholesterol contained in the blood; blood cholesterol levels vary significantly from person to person and are determined by a complex mixture of factors, including cholesterol intake level and the quantity of cholesterol produced by the body.

Blood clot: A network of blood cells and molecules that solidifies in the bloodstream and stops the flow of blood.

Bronchi: The two large tubular airways that connect the air sacs of the lung with the trachea.

Bronchioles: The smallest airways within the lungs that connect the air sacs of the lung with the bronchi.

Bronchodilators: A group of drugs that widen the airways in the lungs and are used to treat a variety of conditions in which the flow of air into the lungs is obstructed or reduced.

C

Calcium channel blockers: Medications that block the movement of calcium across the cell membranes of arterial muscle cells, with the result that the muscles relax and blood pressure decreases.

Cardiopulmonary resuscitation (CPR): An emergency procdure used to treat someone who is not breathing or whose heart has stopped beating by applying a combination of external cardiac massage and rescue breathing.

Cardiovascular diseases: Diseases of the heart and blood vessels.

145

Carotids: Arteries in the neck leading to the brain.

Chemotherapy: Treatment involving the use of drugs or other medication designed to kill or reduce the growth rae of cancer cells.

Cholesterol: A fat-like substance found in animal foods and also manufactured by the body. Cholesterol is essential to nerve and brain cell function and to the synthesis of sex hormones and is also a component of bile acids used to aid fat digestion. It is also a part of atherosclerotic plaques that accumulate on artery walls.

Chronic bronchitis: A persistent inflammation of the bronchial tubes accompanied by the coughing up of excess mucus that extends for an interval of 3 or more months each year for at least 2 consecutive years.

Colonoscopy: A procedure that involves viewing the inside of the entire colon, usually for diagnostic purposes, by means of a long, flexible instrument called a colonoscope.

Congenital heart disease: Structural abnormalities of the heart that occur during development within the fetus.

Congestive heart failure: Ineffective pumping of both sides of the heart, leading to a buildup of fluid within the tissues of the body.

Contact inhibition: A natural feedback mechanism whereby a normal cell stops growing when it touches a surrounding cell.

Contraindications: Factors in a person's physical condition that make it unwise to pursue a certain line of treatment.

Coronary arteries: The arteries lying on the surface of the heart muscle that provide the heart with its blood supply.

Corticosteroids: Hormonal preparations that help to diminish inflammation; they are used to treat a variety of conditions, including asthma.

Cystic fibrosis: A genetically inherited disease characterized by excessive mucus production by the lining of the bronchial tubes and an inability to digest fats; although a variety of treatments are now available, cystic fibrosis remains a serious and ultimately life-threatening disease.

D

Diabetes: A disorder characterized by abnormally high levels of glucose (sugar) in the blood resulting from the failure of the pancreas to produce a sufficient supply of insulin, the hormone responsible for the conversion of glucose into a form usable by the cells of the body.

Diastolic: The filling phase of the heartbeat, reflected in the second or lower number of the blood pressure reading.

Dietary cholesterol: Cholesterol contained in the diet; cholesterol intake.

Diuretics: Medications that allow the kidneys to excrete more salt and, consequently, more water than usual.

E

Electrocardiogram (EKG): The electrical tracing of the heartbeat.

Embolism: A blockage of an artery caused by a clump of material (embolus) circulating in the bloodstream; embolisms are named after the affected part of the body; cerebral embolisms affect the blood supply to the brain, pulmonary embolisms affect the blood supply to the lungs, and so forth.

Emphysema: A severe lung disorder characterized by the gradual destruction of the tiny air sacs in the lung (alveoli) and a reduction in elasticity of lung tissue that impairs the lung's efficiency; the major symptom is a marked shortness of breath.

Endometrium: The lining of the uterus.

Esophagus: The tubular structure located immediately behind the windpipe (trachea) that connects the mouth and the stomach.

Estrogen: A female sex hormone responsible for secondary sex characteristics and for providing a suitable environment for conception during the menstrual cycle.

F

Fatty acids: Chemical compounds containing carbon, hydrogen, and oxygen. They form part of the triglycerides in food and in the body and can be saturated, polyunsaturated, or monounsaturated.

Fibrosis: Any overgrowth of scar or connective tissue, particularly one which replaces normal surrounding tissue; such overgrowths can significantly impair vital body functions when they occur in specialized organs such as the lungs.

G

Glucose: A simple sugar that is the major energy source for the cells of the body.

Growth factor: Abnormal proteins that ignore natural feedback and stimulate cells to continue to grow and multiply, resulting in a tumor.

H

HDL cholesterol: The so-called good cholesterol, a lipid compound that contains cholesterol removed from the arteries; high HDL cholesterol levels reduce the risk of heart disease.

Heart failure: Ineffective pumping of one side of the heart leading to a buildup of fluid within the tissues of the body, commonly in the lungs and the feet.

Hematocrit: Shorthand label for a measurement of the number of red blood cells in a blood sample as determined by a procedure involving a specialized centrifuge known as a hematocrit; also known as hematocrit value.

Hemorrhage: Uncontrollable, excessive bleeding.

Hodgkin's disease: A cancer of the lymph tissue (lymph nodes, spleen) in which the malignant cells reproduce rapidly and cause a swelling of the lymph nodes, typically those in the neck or armpits.

Hypercalcemia: An abnormally high level of calcium in the blood.

Hyperlipidemia: Elevated levels of fats in the blood.

Hypertension: The medical term for abnormally high blood pressure.

I

Influenza: A viral respiratory infection popularly known as the "flu"; the symptoms of influenza include fever, chills, headache, muscle ache, loss of appetite, and general weakness.

Insulin: A hormone produced by the pancreas in varying amounts depending on the level of blood sugar; it promotes the absorption and use of glucose by the liver and muscles.

Ischemia: A chronic reduction in blood supply that results in the inability of the affected organ to function in a normal manner.

L

Larynx: Voice box; the area surrounding and including the vocal cords.

LDL cholesterol: The so-called bad cholesterol; a form of cholesterol that is deposited on the walls of arteries, contributing to the process of atherosclerosis and thus the risk of heart disease.

Lipid: A class of fatty substances that are insoluble in water, transported throughout the body by the blood, and are one of the body's important sources of food energy; the more important types of lipids include triglycerides (the principal component of body fat) and sterols such as cholesterol.

Lipoproteins: A class of proteins found in the blood that consist of a simple protein combined with a lipid (fatty substances that are otherwise insoluble in water). They are transported throughout the body by the blood.

Lumpectomy: The removal of a lump, usually referring to the removal of a cancerous lump in a woman's breast without removing the breast.

Lymph nodes: Glands that produce and filter lymph, a clear fluid containing antibodies and white blood cells that circulates through the lymphatic system.

Lytic drug: Medication used in the treatment of a heart attack that dissolves (or lyses) recently formed blood clots.

M

Malignant or cancerous cells: A tumor that is not confined and has a tendency to infiltrate normal tissue and metastasize.

Mastectomy: Surgical removal of the breast tissue.

Maximum heart rate: The number obtained by subtracting your age from 220; the resulting difference is defined as the maximum heart rate (in number of beats per minute) and should not be exceeded.

Melanoma: A skin cancer derived from the pigment-secreting cells in the skin; it is highly malignant and may cause death.

Metastasis: The movement of malignant cells to, and proliferation at, body sites other than those at which the tissue of origin was located.

Monounsaturated fat: These are one of two types of unsaturated fats, fats that contain less than the maximum possible amount of hydrogen. Monounsaturated fats contain one less hydrogen bond than the maximum number possible.

Myocardial infarction: The medical term for a heart attack.

Myocardium: Heart muscle.

O

Osteoporosis: A disturbance of bone metabolism in which the bone mass decreases and the bones become more fragile.

P

Pap smear: A test designed to detect abnormal changes in a small sample containing cells from the surface of the cervix (the neck of the uterus).

Parathyroid hormone: A hormone produced by the parathyroid glands, located in the neck, that helps to control the level of calcium in the blood.

Phlegm: Mucus, especially in excessive amounts, produced by the cells lining the bronchial tree and excreted by the respiratory system.

Plaque: A raised area on the inner lining of the artery wall consisting of low-density lipoproteins, cellular debris, cholesterol, and sometimes calium; such deposits tend to form in areas of relatively turbulent blood flow, e.g., the coronary arteries.

Polyunsaturated fats: One of two types of unsaturated fats, fats that contain less than the maximum possible amount of hydrogen. Polyunsaturated fats contain two or more fewer hydrogen bonds than the maximum possible.

Proctosigmoidoscopy: A procedure that involves the visual inspection of the lower (sigmoid) colon and rectum via a viewing instrument known as a proctosigmoidoscope.

Progesterone: A female sex hormone that plays a major role in the menstrual cycle.

Pulmonary embolism: A blood clot that travels to the lung.

Pulmonary function tests: Breathing tests that measure several aspects of the respiratory cycle, including the amount of air exhaled and the force of expiration, to help determine if there is any impediment to the flow of air to or from the lungs.

R

Radiation treatments: The use of X rays to treat cancer.

Resorption: The organic breaking down of a structure into parts and the assimilation of those parts for a different use.

Rheumatic heart disease: Damage done to the heart, usually to the valves, by the inflammation associated with rheumatic fever.

Rubella: A viral infection, also known as German measles, whose usual symptoms are a mild fever and skin rash that lasts for several days, then disappears.

S

Saturated fat: A type of fatty acid containing the maximum possible amount of hydrogen; palm oil, coconut oil, and most animal fats are highly saturated fats.

Sigmoidoscopy: A screening procedure that involves viewing the last 50 centimeters of the colon with a short, flexible viewing device called a sigmoidoscope.

Squamous cell cancer (carcinoma): A form of skin cancer that usually takes the form of red, scaly patches or lesions on the lips, face, or tips of the ears.

Strep infection: An infection caused by the streptococcus organism.

Stroke: Damage to part of the brain caused by interruption to its blood supply, resulting in physical or mental impairment or even death.

Systolic: The pumping phase of the heartbeat, reflected in the first or higher number of the blood pressure reading.

T

Theophylline: A bronchodilator that is primarily used in the treatment of asthma.

Thrombus: A blood clot that forms within a blood vessel.

Trachea: The windpipe that connects the airways of the lungs to the mouth.

Type A: A pattern of behavior characterized by overwork, hostility, inability to relax, and a tendency to hurry.

U

Uterine cervix: The neck of the uterus, which protrudes into the top of the vaginal canal.

V

Ventricle: Pumping chamber in the heart.

Notes

CHAPTER 1

1. *The 1989 Information Please Almanac*, 42d ed. (Boston: Houghton Mifflin Company, 1989), 794.
2. *Statistical Abstract of the United States, 1990*, 110th ed., (Washington, DC: Government Printing Office, 1990).
3. C. Popescu, "The Good News About America's Health," *Changing Times*, October 1988, 117.
4. American Heart Association, *Fact Sheet on Heart Attack, Stroke and Risk Factors*, Pamphlet no. 51-1011 (COM) (November 1988), 11-88-350M.
5. Eugene Braunwald, *Harrison's Principles in Internal Medicine*, 11th ed. (New York: McGraw-Hill, 1987), 985.
6. American Heart Association, *The Heart and Blood Vessels*, Pamphlet no. 50-006-A (Rev. 80) 73-83-2.65MM, 10-84-500M, 11.
7. Braunwald, p. 982.
8. Steering Committee of the Physician's Health Study Research Group, "Final Report on the Aspirin Component of the Ongoing Physician's Health Study," *New England Journal of Medicine* 321, no. 3 (July 1989): 129–135.
9. Braunwald, p. 984.
10. *Internal Medicine News*, (15–31 January 1990): 2.
11. For a more in-depth discussion of smoking, see Richard G. Schlaadt, *Wellness: Tobacco & Health* (Guilford, CT: The Dushkin Publishing Group, 1992).
12. "The 1988 Report of the Joint National Committee on Detection, Evaluation and Treatment of High Blood Pressure," *Archives of Internal Medicine* 148 (May 1988): 1023–1038.
13. "Hypertension, Prevalence, and the Status of Awareness, Treatment and Control in the United States: Final Report of the Subcommittee on Definition and Prevalence of the 1984 Joint Committee," *Hypertension* 7, no. 3 (May/June 1985): 457–468.
14. Braunwald, p. 1018.
15. Braunwald, p. 1018.
16. American Heart Association, *Heart and Stroke Facts*, Pamphlet no. 55-0376 (COM) 11-89-135M, 89 08 04 A (1990), 18.
17. "Report: National Cholesterol Education Program Expert Panel on Detection, Evaluation and Treatment of High Blood

Cholesterol in Adults," *Archives of Internal Medicine* 148 (January 1988): 36–69.

18. "Report: National Cholesterol Education Program Expert Panel on Detection, Evaluation and Treatment of High Blood Cholesterol in Adults," pp. 36–69.

19. Braunwald, p. 1019.

20. S. Harris, "Exercise and the Heart: Report of the U.S. Preventive Services Task Force," *Primary Cardiology* 16, no. 3 (March 1990): 41–50.

21. Harris, p. 53.

22. Braunwald, p. 1019.

23. Braunwald, pp. 1832–1834.

24. Braunwald, p. 1019.

CHAPTER 2

1. *Heart and Stroke Facts.*

2. American Heart Association, Pamphlet no. 50-052-D 86-88-1.351MM 11-89-600M 860114A.

3. *Heart and Stroke Facts,* p. 19.

4. "Report of the Joint National Committee on Detection, Evaluation and Treatment of High Blood Pressure," p. 1033.

5. *Heart and Stroke Facts,* p. 19.

6. American Heart Association, *Strokes, A Guide for the Family,* Pamphlet no. 50-025-B, 81-82-300M, 10-83-200M.

CHAPTER 3

1. American Cancer Society, *Cancer Facts and Figures,* Pamphlet 90-425M no. 5008-LE (1990).

2. *Cancer Journal for Clinicians* 40, no. 1 (January/February 1990): 9.

3. Braunwald, p. 1115.

4. Braunwald, p. 1116.

5. Goroll, *Primary Care Medicine* (Philadelphia: J. B. Lippincott, 1981), 176–177.

6. Braunwald, p. 1116.

7. Braunwald, p. 857.

8. Department of Health and Human Services, Public Health Service, Centers for Disease Control, Office of Smoking and Health, "Passive Smoking: A Report of the Surgeon General" (Rockville, MD: 1986), 19.

9. *Cancer Facts and Figures,* p. 20.
10. *Cancer Journal for Clinicians* 40, no. 1, p. 9.
11. *Cancer Facts and Figures,* p. 10.
12. Braunwald, p. 1571.
13. Eugene Braunwald, *Harrison's Principles in Internal Medicine* 12th ed. (New York: McGraw-Hill, 1987), 1619.
14. Braunwald, 11th ed., p. 1567.
15. Braunwald, 12th ed., p. 1615.
16. Braunwald, 12th ed., p. 1615.
17. *Cancer Facts and Figures,* p. 9.
18. American Cancer Society, *Colorectal Cancer—Go for Early Detection,* Pamphlet no. 83-2MM Rev. 4/89 2051-LE.
19. American Cancer Society, *Facts on Colorectal Cancer,* Pamphlet no. 88-500M-No. 2004-LE, 7.
20. *Facts on Colorectal Cancer.*
21. *Cancer Facts and Figures.*
22. *Cancer Facts and Figures.*
23. *Cancer Facts and Figures,* p. 13.
24. Braunwald, 12th ed., p. 1630.
25. Braunwald, 12th ed., p. 1631.
26. Braunwald, 11th ed., p. 1541.
27. *Cancer Facts and Figures,* p. 14.
28. Braunwald, 11th ed.
29. *Cancer Facts and Figures,* p. 14.
30. *Cancer Facts and Figures,* p. 15.
31. Braunwald, 12th ed., p. 1637.
32. *Cancer Facts and Figures,* p. 18.
33. *Cancer Facts and Figures,* p. 18.
34. American Cancer Society, *Taking Control,* Pamphlet no. 85-5MM-Rev. 5/87-No. 2019.05.

CHAPTER 4

1. American Lung Association, *Emphysema: Facts About Your Lungs,* Pamphlet (April 1986), 1.
2. Braunwald, 11th ed., p. 857.
3. Braunwald, 11th ed., p. 1068.
4. Braunwald, 11th ed., p. 1066.
5. American Lung Association, *Asthma: Facts About Your Lungs,* Pamphlet no. 0052 5/84, 3.
6. American Lung Association, *Facts About Flu,* Pamphlet no. 9/88.

CHAPTER 5

1. N. Stone, "Preventive Cardiology: The Physican's Role in Dietary Fat Counseling," *RX Nutrition* (Little Falls, NJ: Health Learning Systems), 245.
2. Stone, p. 248.
3. "Report to the National Cholesterol Education Program Expert Panel on Detection, Evaluation and Treatment of High Blood Cholesterol in Adults," *Archives of Internal Medicine* 148 (January 1989): 36–69.
4. Braunwald, 11th ed., p. 1021.
5. Department of Health and Human Services, *Non-Insulin Dependent Diabetes,* Publication no. 87-241 (March 1987): 1.
6. *Non-Insulin Dependent Diabetes,* p. 3.
7. *Non-Insulin Dependent Diabetes,* p. 4.
8. *Non-Insulin Dependent Diabetes,* p. 4.
9. Trachtenbarg, "Treatment of Osteoporosis," *Post-Graduate Medicine* 87, no. 4 (March 1990): 263.
10. Braunwald, 11th ed., p. 1891.
11. Don Gambrell, "Use of Progesterone Challenge Test to Reduce the Risk of Endometrial Cancer," *Obstetrics and Gynecology* 55:6 (June 1980): 732–739.

CHAPTER 6

1. *Statistical Abstract of the United States, 1990,* 110th ed., (Washington, DC: Government Printing Office, 1990).
2. E. Monsen, "Symposium Proceedings: Good Health in Practice," *RX Nutrition:* 2.
3. Monsen, pp. 5–6.
4. W. Conner, "Dietary Fiber: Nostrum or Critical Nutrient?" *New England Journal of Medicine* 322, no. 3 (January 1990): 193–195.
5. R. Butrum, "National Cancer Institute Dietary Guidelines: Rationale," *American Journal of Clinical Nutrition* 48 (1988): 888–895.
6. Trachtenbarg, pp. 263–270.
7. Monsen, pp. 5–6.
8. Monsen, p. 13.
9. Harris, pp. 41–50.
10. American Cancer Society, *Danger,* Pamphlet no. 78-(1MM)-No. 2053-LE.

Resources

BOOKS

Aloia, John F., M.D. *Osteoporosis: A Guide to Prevention and Treatment*. Champaign, IL: Leisure Press, 1989.

This debilitating disease that weakens bones and causes pain, disability, and deformity is discussed in comprehensive detail in this book. The author shows who is most likely to get osteoporosis and why, factors that contribute to getting the disease, the role of calcium and other dietary supplements, estrogen and exercise therapy, and the most effective methods of pain reduction.

Brody, Jane. *The New York Times Guide to Personal Health*. New York: The New York Times Book Co., 1982.

Based on Jane Brody's award-winning and immensely popular "Personal Health" columns from the *New York Times*, this book helps the reader take charge of his or her health. It teaches how to stay healthy, how to participate in medical care, what to do when things go wrong, how to avoid unnecessary and expensive treatment, and how to get better care from doctors. Fifteen sections include: nutrition, exercise, emotional health, environmental health effects, common serious illnesses, and more.

Connor, Sonia L., and William E. Connor. *The New American Diet*. New York: Simon & Schuster, 1989.

This book discusses the information available on cholesterol and heart disease, which establishes the necessary background for the authors' approach to dietary regulation of fats through the CSFI, or Cholesterol Saturation Fat Index. The book includes recipes and guides for long-term dietary fat reduction.

Cooper, Kenneth H., M.D. *Controlling Cholesterol: Dr. Kenneth H. Cooper's Preventive Medicine Program*. New York: Bantam, 1988.

The author presents a program for identifying personal risk for heart disease, controlling cholesterol levels, and reducing risk of heart disease. Also discussed are diet, alcohol, smoking, exercise, stress, birth-control pills, fish oil, fiber, how to obtain an accurate blood-cholesterol profile, and other topics.

Cooper, Kenneth H., M.D. *Preventing Osteoporosis*. New York: Bantam Books, 1989.

Dr. Cooper shows that osteoporosis is not just a disease of the elderly or of women. He discusses how to increase bone density and strengthen brittle bones, exactly who in our population is likely to develop osteoporosis, the factors that cause the disease, and possible cures. The author provides charts, exercises, recipes, and information on calcium supplements and estrogen replacement to aid in treatment.

Dreher, Henry. *Your Defense Against Cancer: The Complete Guide to Cancer Prevention*. New York: Harper & Row, 1988.

This book provides extensive information on how to avoid known cancer-causing agents in food, water, air and a host of other environmental factors to which we are exposed every day. A 24-page section of the book is dedicated to the influence of smoking on cancer. This chapter, entitled *Smoking: The Most Dangerous Habit*, presents the known facts of nicotine's powerful effect as a drug, examines what happens when smokers smoke, and presents a detailed discussion on how to become a nonsmoker.

Glenn, Jim. *Colds and Coughs*. Springhouse, PA: Springhouse Corporation, 1986.

The common cold, influenza, and their associated symptoms of sore throats, fever, headache, and stuffy nose are covered in this book. Glenn also explains how the body fights infection, how to avoid colds and influenza viruses, what to do when a cold strikes, the doctor's role in diagnosis and treatment, the complications that can develop from colds and flu, and more.

Howard, Elliot J., M.D., with Susan A. Roth. *Health Risks*. Tucson, AZ: The Body Press, 1986.

The author provides a detailed discussion of the risk factors and life-style changes that reduce the likelihood of developing cancer, heart disease, stroke, osteoporosis, diabetes, and stress-related problems.

Jovanovic, Lois, M.D., June Biermann, and Barbara Toohey. *The Diabetic Woman*. Los Angeles: J. P. Tarcher, distributed by St. Martin's Press, 1987.

This practical, personal, often humorous guide addresses the special problems and needs of women who are diabetic. The book is organized

153

according to the specific stages of a woman's life, from childhood to maturity. Information is also provided on diabetes and losing weight, menopause, energy level, pregnancy, sex life, sports and exercise, and more.

Keet, Robert B., M.D., and Mary Nelson, M.S. *The Medical Marketplace.* Santa Cruz, CA: Network Publications, 1985.

Keet and Nelson present information and checklists to help you plan your health care and make wise health decisions. They cover choosing a physician, emergency care, medications, surgery, and other topics.

Kunz, Jeffery R.M., and Asher J. Finkel, M.D., eds. *The American Medical Association Family Medical Guide.* New York: Random House, 1987.

This comprehensive guide covers topics ranging from maintaining a healthy body to caring for the ill. A section on symptoms and self-diagnosis uses flowcharts to help the reader track down the possible significance of a particular symptom or set of symptoms, and another section provides explanations of diseases and disorders.

Phillips, Robert, H. *Coping with Osteoarthritis.* New York: Avery Publishing Group, 1989.

Written in an easy-to-read style, this handbook provides effective strategies and techniques for dealing with the physical and emotional problems of osteoarthritis. The disease is defined, and diagnosis and treatment are discussed.

Roth, Eli M., and Sandra L. Streicher. *Good Cholesterol, Bad Cholesterol.* Rocklin, CA: Prima Publishing and Communications, 1989.

So-called good cholesterol (HDL) and bad cholesterol (LDL) are defined and explained in this book. The authors teach how to read food labels to determine the amounts of fats in food, how to increase the intake of HDL (good) cholesterol, and how to reduce LDL cholesterol levels through foods and medications when necessary. Cooking ideas for low-cholesterol meals are also provided.

The New Illustrated Family Medical and Health Guide. By the Editors of Consumer's Guide. Lincolnwood, IL: Publications International, Inc., 1991.

This book covers a wide variety of health and medical topics to help readers make the best decisions about personal and family health-care needs. It provides information to help choose the appropriate doctor, stay healthy, prevent illness, and be better informed on med-ical and health-care systems, tests, and treatments. Also included are nutrition and life-style guidelines and sections on recognizing and coping with common symptoms, infectious diseases, and inherited conditions.

Whitaker, Julian, M., M.D. *Reversing Heart Disease.* New York: Warner Books, 1985.

The author discusses an alternative therapy to traditional medicine for reducing the chances of developing heart disease and repairing damage already done to the circulatory system. Whitaker presents clinical studies and other information to show that a program of diet and exercise can lower cholesterol, reduce weight, and thus lower the risk factors of heart disease and reduce, if not eliminate, the need for heart-disease medications.

NEWSLETTERS

ACSH News and Views is published 5 times a year by the American Council on Science and Health, a nonprofit educational association. The newsletter discusses topics related to food, chemicals, the environment, and health. A one-year subscription is $15. Write to ACSH News and Views, 1995 Broadway, New York, NY 10023-5860, or call (212) 362-7044.

Consumer Reports Health Letter is published monthly by Consumers Union of the United States, a nonprofit organization that provides information and advice on products, services, health, and personal finance. A one-year subscription is $24; a 2-year one costs $38. Write to the Subscription Director, Consumer Reports Health Letter, Box 56356, Boulder, CO 80322-6356, or call (800) 274-8370.

FDA Consumer is published 10 times a year by the Food and Drug Administration, U.S. Public Health Service, Department of Health and Human Services. This magazine provides 6 feature articles on a wide range of topics related to health, health care and health-care products, medicines, medical technologies, diseases, food safety, and so on. Regular columns include brief updates; an AIDS page; investigators' reports, exposing fraud; and summaries of court actions, which provide information on drugs, medical services and devices, foods, and even veterinary drugs that have come under the scrutiny of the law.

Harvard Health Letter is published monthly as a nonprofit service by the Department of Continuing Education, Harvard Medical School, in association with Harvard University Press. The letter has the goal of interpreting health information for general readers in a timely and accurate fashion. A one-year subscription is $21. Write to Harvard Medical School Letter, 79 Garden Street, Cambridge, MA 02138, or call customer service at (617) 495-3975.

Healthline is published monthly by Healthline Publishing, Inc. The letter is intended to educate readers about ways to help themselves avoid illness and to live longer, healthier lives. A one-year subscription is $19, or $34 for 2 years. Write to Healthline, The C.V. Mosby Company, 11830 Westline Industrial Drive, St. Louis, MO 63146-3318, or call (800) 325-4177 (ext. 351).

Johns Hopkins Medical Letter, Health After 50, is published monthly by Medletter Associates, Inc., and covers a variety of topics related to healthful living. A one-year subscription is $20. Write to Johns Hopkins Medical Letter, P.O. Box 420179, Palm Coast, FL 32142.

Lahey Clinic Health Letter is published monthly to bring readers timely, relevant information about important medical issues. Continuing topics include general healthfulness, natural and processed foods, depression, exercise, alcohol, prescription medicine therapy, and major diseases. A one-year subscription is $18. Write to Lahey Clinic Health Letter, Subscription Department, P.O. Box 541, Burlington, MA 01805.

University of California, Berkeley Wellness Letter is published monthly and covers many topics, including nutrition, fitness, and stress management. A one-year subscription is $20. Write to University of California, Berkeley Wellness Letter, P.O. Box 420148, Palm Coast, FL 32142.

PERIODICALS

American Health Magazine: Fitness of Body and Mind is published 10 times a year and covers many aspects of physical and mental well-being. In addition to feature articles, ongoing departments include Nutrition News, Fitness Reports, Mind/Body News, Family Report, Family Pet, and more. A one-year subscription is $14.95. Write to American Health: Fitness of Body and Mind, P.O. Box 3015, Harlan, IA 51537-3015.

Current Health 2: The Continuing Guide to Health Education is published monthly from September through May. Each issue contains a feature article plus a number of shorter pieces on topics such as drugs, psychology, your personal health, disease, and nutrition. For subscription information, contact *Current Health 2*, Publication and Subscription Offices, Field Publications, 4343 Equity Drive, Columbus, Ohio 43228.

Diabetes Self-Management is published bimonthly by R. A. Rapaport Publishing, Inc. Feature articles cover every aspect of living with and managing diabetes, including nutrition, exercise, footware, and other topics for diabetic patients. Regular departments include Women and Diabetes, Supermarket Smarts, Sports and Fitness, and the Diabetes Quiz. A one-year subscription costs $18. Write R. A. Rapaport Publishing, Inc., 150 West 22d Street, New York, NY 10011.

In Health Magazine is published 6 times a year and provides articles on a number of health issues. In addition to recipes and practical nutritional tips, the magazine regularly includes self-help resources for consumers. A one-year subscription is $18. Write to In Health, P.O. Box 52431, Boulder, CO 80321-2431.

Living with Allergies is published once a year by the American Allergy Association (AAA). The publication includes articles on maintaining an allergen-free diet and environment, allergen-free recipes, book reviews, and pollen data. The price is $15 and includes membership in the American Allergy Association. Write AAA, P.O. Box 7273, Menlo Park, CA 94026, or call (415) 322-1663.

Priorities: For Long Life & Good Health is published quarterly by the American Council of Science and Health, Inc., (ACSH), a nonprofit consumer education association concerned with nutrition, chemicals, life-style factors, the environment, and human health. General individual membership to ACSH, which includes a subscription to Priorities, costs $25 a year. Write to the Subscription Department, Priorities, 1995 Broadway, 16th Floor, New York, NY 10023-5860.

HOTLINES

Allergy/Asthma Hotline, (800) 822-2762. Call this number for information on allergies and asthma and to help locate a medical specialist in your area. This number is sponsored by the American Academy of Allergy and Immunology in Milwaukee, Wisconsin.

American Diabetes Association, (800) ADA-DISC. Staff members will answer general questions about diabetes, risk factors, and symptoms. Free literature and a free quarterly newsletter, *Diabetes,* will be sent upon request. Service is available from 8:30 A.M. to 5:00 P.M., Eastern Standard Time, Monday through Friday.

American Dietetic Association, (800) 877-1600. The American Dietetic Association (ADA) is the major professional organization for the dietetic profession. The ADA will answer questions and provide information related to foods and nutrition.

Arthritis Foundation Information Line, (800) 283-7800. This organization will provide information, referrals, pamphlets, brochures, and other publications upon request. It also collects and disseminates information on arthritis and related diseases and works to further educate the public as well as health-care professionals on these disorders.

Cancer Information Service, (800) 4-CANCER. This hotline is funded by the National Cancer Institute and is staffed both by professionals and volunteers. They will answer questions on causes of cancer, prevention, detection, and treatment and will counsel about cancer-related problems. Literature is available upon request, and referrals are made to cancer support groups, treatment facilities, and transportation services. The service is available from 9:00 A.M. to 10:00 P.M., Monday through Friday, and from 10:00 A.M. to 6 P.M. Saturday, Eastern Standard Time.

National Cancer Institute Cancer Information Line, (800) 638-6694 nationwide; (800) 492-6600 in Maryland. It offers free pamphlets about the causes, prevention, detection, diagnosis, and treatment of cancer to patients, families, and friends. It also provides referrals to cancer centers in 23 states. Daily hours are 8 A.M. to midnight, Eastern Standard Time.

National Health Information Center, Department of Health and Human Services, (800) 336-4797; in Maryland, call (301) 656-4167. Operated by the Office of Disease Prevention and Health Promotion, this information and referral center's trained personnel will direct you to the organization or government agency that can assist you with your health questions about high blood pressure, cancer, fitness, or any other topic. Its hours are 9:00 A.M. to 5:00 P.M., Eastern Standard Time, Monday through Friday.

Tel-Med is a free telephone service provided in many cities. You can call and ask for a specific audiotape number and have the health message played for you over the telephone. There are over 300 medical topics to choose from, including topics related to maintaining a healthy life-style, and many states provide toll-free numbers for this service. Call your local information operator to find the nearest Tel-Med office, or write to Tel-Med, Box 970, Colton, CA 92324.

VIDEOTAPES

The following video programs related to wellness topics can be ordered from the National Wellness Institute, Inc., South Hall, 1319 Fremont Street, Stevens Point, WI 54481. Write to request format, price, and ordering information.

Living with High Blood Pressure is hosted by Arthur Ashe, the legendary tennis professional and a heart-attack victim. This video will help you learn how heredity and life-style affect your blood pressure, how to understand clearly the disease, and how to live with high blood pressure.

Lower Your Cholesterol Now! is an upbeat, informative, and practical video. Dietitionist Leni Reed provides facts and advice on how to make wise nutritional choices to lower your intake of calories, saturated fats, and cholesterol in your diet.

GOVERNMENT, CONSUMER, AND ADVOCACY GROUPS

American Allergy Association (AAA), P.O. Box 7273, Menlo Park, CA 94026, (415) 322-1663
    The AAA consists of participants who are allergy patients and others interested in the problems created by allergies. The group disseminates information on diet, environmental control, and other influences causing allergic reactions. It publishes *Living with Allergies* annually and also pamphlets on allergies.
American Cancer Society (ACS), 1599 Cliffs Road, Atlanta, GA 30329, (404) 320-3333

The ACS supports education and research in cancer prevention, diagnosis, detection, and treatment, including the health effects of tobacco and alcohol use, stress, genetic inheritance, and a host of other cancer-causing suspects. It provides special services to cancer patients and sponsors Reach to Recovery, Can-Surmount, and I Can Cope.

American Heart Association (AHA), 720 Greenville Avenue, Dallas, TX 75231, (214) 373-6300

The AHA supports research, education, and community-service programs with the goal of reducing premature death and disability from stroke and cardiovascular disease. It publishes several books, periodicals, and pamphlets yearly that are related to management of a healthy heart. State branches of the AHA can be located through directory information.

American Lung Association (ALA), 1740 Broadway, New York, NY 10019, (212) 315-8700

Membership includes a federation of state and local associations of physicians, nurses, and laypeople interested in the prevention and control of lung disease. The ALA works with other organizations in planning and conducting programs in community services; public, professional, and patient education; and research. It makes policy recommendations regarding medical care of patients with respiratory diseases, occupational health, hazards of smoking, and air conservation. The ALA is financed by the annual Christmas Seal Campaign and other fund-raising activities.

Arthritis Foundation (AF), 1312 Spring Street, NW Atlanta, GA 30309, (404) 872-7100

Founded in 1948, the Arthritis Foundation seeks to discover the causes of and improve the methods for treatment and prevention of arthritis and other rheumatic diseases. The foundation provides information and pamphlets to the layperson on subjects concerned with arthritis and publishes *Arthritis Today* bimonthly, which includes book reviews, research reports, and self-help tips.

Arthritis Information Clearinghouse (AIC), P.O. Box 34427, Bethesda, MD 20034, (301) 881-9411

The AIC catalogs and disseminates information about arthritis and related diseases from a variety of sources. It serves as an information exchange for individuals and organizations involved in public, professional, and patient education and refers personal queries from patients to the Arthritis Foundation.

Asthma and Allergy Foundation of America (AAFA), 1717 Massachusetts Avenue, Suite 305, Washington, DC 20036, (202) 265-0265

The AAFA is a national voluntary health agency that seeks to solve the health problems created by allergic reactions to foods, pollens, drugs, molds, and insect bites. The foundation provides information and educational materials to the public and to health professionals. The AAFA publishes *ADVANCE* bimonthly and other bulletins.

Cancer Information Clearinghouse, National Cancer Institute, Office of Cancer Communications, 9000 Rockville Pike, Building 31, Room 10A18, Bethesda, MD 20205, (301) 496-4070

This organization collects and disseminates information on public, patient, and professional cancer-education materials to individuals, organizations, and health-care professionals.

Centers for Disease Control (CDC), Dr. Robert Waller, Project Coordinator, 1600 Cliffs Park, Executive Plaza, Building 26, Mail Stop E25, Atlanta, GA 30333, (404) 639-3311

This main telephone number connects you with an operator who will then direct you to the specific information laboratory for the answers you seek regarding hepatitis, AIDS, venereal diseases, and so on. You may also be referred to someone in the Public Inquiry department who will in turn handle your inquiry for a specific disease.

High Blood Pressure Information Center (HBPIC), 120/80 National Institutes of Health, Bethesda, MD 20205, (301) 652-7700

The HBPIC provides information on the detection, diagnosis, and management of high blood pressure to consumers and health professionals. The center identifies, collects, organizes, and disseminates information in many formats. Its sources are monographs, journals, newsletters, newspapers, reports, audiovisuals, brochures, posters, and contacts with other health agencies and clearinghouses. It also provides reference and referral services, consultants, a speaker's register, packets, searches on the center's data base, and resources of and referrals to other libraries and clearinghouses.

National Clearinghouse for Human Genetic Diseases, 805 15th Street, Suite 500, Washington, DC 20005, (202) 842-7617

This clearinghouse provides information on human genetics and genetic diseases for both patients and health-care workers, and it also reviews existing curricular materials on genetic education.

National Diabetes Information Clearinghouse, 805 15th Street, NW, Suite 500, Washington, DC 20005, (202) 842-7630

This clearinghouse collects and disseminates information on patient-education materials and coordinates the development of materials and programs for diabetes education.

National Foundation for Asthma (NFA), P.O. Box 30069, Tucson, AZ 85751, (602) 323-6046

This agency provides medical and social rehabilitation care for chronic asthma patients and offers emergency-room treatment and ambulatory pulmonary care. The NFA also operates out-patient clinical care for the treatment of asthma, allergies, and other related diseases and provides allergy testing, immunotherapy, and physical therapy for asthma sufferers. The Foundation publishes *Asthma: Fact and Fiction, Weeds 'n Things and Dust 'n Stuff* in addition to handbooks and reports.

ODPHP (Office of Disease Prevention and Health Promotion) National Health Information Center (NHIC), P.O. Box 1133, Washington, DC 20013, (301) 565-4167

This center—funded by the ODPHP, the Public Health Service, and the Department of Health and Human Services—aids consumers and health professionals in locating health information. It publishes several health bulletins and health-information resource booklets as well as health information specifically for women.

Index

20–21, 26; and high blood
pressure, 34, 35, 40, 51
occupational lung diseases, 94
oil, and cholesterol, 112, 113
oral cancer, and smoking, 60
oral contraceptives: and breast
cancer, 66; and risk of heart
attacks, 23, 25; and high blood
pressure, 34, 36, 51; and strokes,
50
osteoporosis: **123**, 125, 126–127; cause
of, 123; diagnosis and symptoms
of, 123–124; prevention and
treatment of, 124–125; risk factors
of, 128

P

PAACT, *see* Patient Advocates for
Advanced Cancer Treatments
pain, *see* chest pain
Pap smear, **73**, 74
parathyroid hormone, **123**
passive smoke, and cancer, 60
Patient Advocates for Advanced
Cancer Treatments (PAACT), 76
pedunculated polyps, 70, 72
phenylpropanolamine (PPA), and
high blood pressure, 53
phlegm, **58**
physical examinations, *see* medical
checkups
plaque, **42**
platelet cells, 45
pneumocystis carinii pneumonia
(PCP), 107
pneumonia: 105, 106, 107, 108;
bacterial, 103, 106; bronchial, 105;
lobar, 105; mycoplasma, 107;
pneumocystis carinii, 107;
prevention of, 108; symptoms of,
108; treatment of, 107; viral,
106–107
polyps, 70–71, 72
polyunsaturated fats, **112**
post-menopausal women: and breast
cancer, 68; and calcium, 132; and
dangers of estrogen therapy, 125,
127–128; and high blood pressure,
35–36; and osteoporosis, 128; and
uterine cancer, 74–75
potassium, loss of, and thiazine
diuretics, 38
PPA, *see* phenylpropanolamine
pregnancy, and high blood pressure,
35
preparation, of food, and lowering
high blood pressure, 52
proctosigmoidoscopy, **69**, 71–72
progesterone, and heart disease, **23**
prostate cancer, 75, 76, 77
psychology, and asthma, 98, 100–103
pulmonary embolism, **23**
pulmonary function tests, **91**

R

race differences: in heart disease, 26;
in high blood pressure, 16, 29; in
life expectancy, 130; in prostate
cancer, 75; in skin cancer, 83; and
risk of stroke, 44
radiation treatments, **57**, 62, 64
rectal, and colon, cancer, 69–73
relaxation, and asthma, 101
resorption, **123**
respiratory system: 85–86; *see also,*
lung cancer; lung disease
rheumatic heart disease, **50**
Rubella, **50**

S

salt: and cancer, 83; and high blood
pressure, 34, 40, 41, 51, 53–54
saturated fat, **111**, 115
self-examination: breast, 64–68; of
testes, 77
serum cholesterol, 114
sessile polyps, 70, 72
sex differences: and incidence of
cancer, 59; and heart attacks, 26,
27; and incidence of high blood
pressure, 16, 29, 32; and risk of
stroke, 44; *see also,* men; women
sigmoidoscopy, **69**
skin cancer: 78–83; causes of, 79–80,
81; prevention of, 80–81, 82; risk
factors for, 83; symptoms of, 81;
treatment of, 82–83
smoking: and aspirin and risk of
heart attack, 14; and cancer,
60–62, 63, 83; and risk of heart
attack, 17–18, 26; and high blood
pressure, 36, 40, 54; and lung
disease, 87, 89, 90, 91, 109;
passive, and cancer, 60; quitting,
and health, 139–140
sodium, *see* salt
spinal deformity: 124; *see also,*
osteoporosis
squamos cell cancer (carcinoma), **78**,
79
"stepped care," for high blood
pressure, 38–39
steroids, 93
stomach ulcer, and chest pain, 10
strep infection, **50**
stress: and risk of heart attacks,
22–23, 26; and high blood
pressure, 34
stroke(s): **17**, 42–45, 47–49; and
aspirin, 14–15; preventing, 49–50;
symptoms of, 45; treatment of,
45–46
sun exposure, and skin cancer, 79–81,
82, 83, 84
sunscreen, and skin cancer, 80–81,
82, 84
support groups: for breast cancer, 66,
76; and family asthma programs,

101–102; lack of, for prostate
cancer, 76
surgery, bypass, 16–17
systolic, **28**, 30, 31, 33

T

target heart rate, and proper
exercise, 137–138
teenagers, and melanoma, 80
testicular carcinoma, 75, 77
theophylline, **92**
thiazine diuretics, 38, 40, 41
thinning, of blood, and aspirin, 13,
15
thrombus, **42**
tobacco, *see* chewing tobacco;
smoking
trachea, **85**, 86
tubolovillous adenomas, 70
tubular polyps, 70
tumor: benign, 56; malignant, 56–57
Type A personality, **23**
Type I diabetes, *see* insulin-dependent
diabetes
Type II diabetes, *see* adult-onset
diabetes

U

ulcers, and chest pain, 10
uterine cancer, 73–75
uterine cervix, **73**

V

vegetable oil, 112, 113
vegetables, and preventing cancer, 83
veins, **5**
ventricle, 3, **5**
ventricular fibrillation, 8
villous adenomas, 70
viral pneumonia, 106–107
virus: influenza, 103, 104, 106;
pneumonia, 106–107
vitamins, and proper diet, 132

W

walking: and blood pressure, 51;
energy expenditure during, 139
water, salt in, and high blood
pressure, 53
weight, *see* obesity
windpipe, *see* trachea
women: and breast cancer, 62–69, 77;
and dangers of estrogen therapy,
125, 127–128; and heart disease,
23, 24, 25, 26, 27, 50; and high
blood pressure, 16, 34, 35–36; and
life expectancy, 1, 130; and
osteoporosis, 128, 132; and
smoking, 62; and uterine cancer,
73–75; *see also,* sex differences

X

X rays, *see* radiation treatments